Healing Wonders of Medicinal Plants in Goa

Dr Suresh Kunkalikar & Carmelito Andrade

Contents

Foreword vii

About the Authors ix

Acknowledgments xi

Who is this book for? xii

How did this book come about? xiii

1. Aloe Vera 15

2. Arjun 17

3. Ash Gourd 19

4. Bael 21

5. Banana 23

6. Betel Leaves 25

7. Betel Nut 27

8. Bitter Gourd 29

9. Black Pepper 31

10. Cathedral bells 33

11. Chaff-flower 35

12. Chaulmoogra Tree 37

13. Chebulic Myrobalan 39

14. Cinnamon 41

15. Cloves 43

16. Coconut 45

17 Cumin 47

18 Custard Apple 49

CONTENTS

19. Edible Stemmed Vine 51

20. Fenugreek 53

21. Flame/Glory Lily 55

22. Garlic 57

23. Ginger 59

24. Green Chiretta 61

25 Himalayan wormwood 63

26 Holy Basil 65

27 Indian Asparagus 67

28. Indian Gooseberry 69

29 Indian devil tree or dita tree 71

30 Indian Hog Plum 73

31 Indian Sarsaparilla 75

32 Indian snakeroot 77

33 Java Plum 79

34 Kokum 81

35 Lime 83

36. Malabar nut 85

37 Mango 87

38 Moringa 89

39 Neem 91

40 Nutmeg 93

41 Onion 95

42 Indian Rennet tree 97

43 Papaya 99

44 Soursop 101

45 Star Fruit 103

46 Sweet Flag.. 105

47 Tamarind 107

48 Tellicherry bark 109

49 Tinospora... 111

50 Toothache tree 113

51 Turmeric 115

52 Wild Karanda 117

Glossary 119

Refrences 122

Foreword

India is rich in biodiversity and a treasure trove for about 8500 medicinal plants. There is a traditional association with the Medicinal Plants (MPs) through the Indian Systems of Medicines (ISMs) like Ayurveda, Siddha, Homeopathy, Sowa - Rigpa, etc. In recent days the acceptance for natural products, herbal medicines have increased due to safety, efficacy, low cost and easy availability in the national and international markets. Presently, MPs are used for production of medicines, nutraceuticals, cosmeceuticals, food supplements, veterinary medicines, animal feed, botanical pesticides etc. In recent days the demand has increased for treatment of dreadful and deadliest diseases like cancer, Alzheimer's, insomnia, diabetes, viral diseases, etc.

However, in the last few decades, rapid urbanization and over-utilization of natural resources has led to resource depletion giving rise to the need for conservation of biodiversity. Like other natural resources, medicinal plants also have been over exploited and the need for conservation of the medicinal plants species was soon recognized by the scientists and experts working in the MAPs sector. The medicinal plants have an exceptional value and there is a certain degree of awareness about the therapeutic properties of the medicinal plant's species due to well-established ISM which has led to significant efforts for conserving the medicinal plants species through various means including establishment of medicinal plants gardens or herbal gardens, Medicinal Plants Conservation Areas (MPCAs), cultivation in agricultural fields, forest areas, etc. Goa is a state on the southwestern coast of India within the Konkan region, geographically separated from the Deccan highlands by the Western Ghats. Goa state is famous for tourism, culture, heritage and historical sites. However, the Goa state has unique medicinal plants and associated traditional knowledge.

The book entitled, 'Healing Wonders of Medicinal Plants in Goa' written by Dr. Suresh Kunkalikar and Mr. Carmelito Andrade is exclusive and provides details of medicinal plants by interacting with local peoples and traditional healers. The book will be useful for the professionals and enthusiasts who are associated with medicinal plants. I congratulate authors and Mr. Maurus Fernandes (Festival Man of Goa) for their efforts.

Prof. (Dr.) Digambar Mokat

Principal Investigator and Regional Director

RCFC-WR (NMPB, Ministry of Ayush, GoI)

Department of Botany

Savitribai Phule Pune University, Pune 411 007

It is a privilege to present this foreword to a volume dedicated to the medicinal plants of Goa, a work that integrates ethnobotanical knowledge with contemporary scientific perspectives. This book stands as both a scholarly contribution and a tribute to Festacar Marius Fernandes, whose enduring commitment to the cultural preservation of Goa for the past quarter of a century continues to inspire meaningful academic and community engagement.

It is my hope that this volume will serve not only as a reference for researchers and students, but also as a tool for conservation, awareness and future exploration of Goa's rich ethnobotanical landscape.

Dr. Gwendolyn de Ornelas

Loutolim, Goa

About the Authors

Dr. Suresh Kunkalikar

Dr. Suresh Kunkalikar, born and brought up in the village of Goa, spent his childhood amid plantations of areca nuts, coconuts, mangoes, pineapples, and cashews, getting knowledge in agriculture. Inspired by the love for nature and agriculture, Dr. Kunkalikar joined the University of Agriculture at Dharwad and completed his Ph.D. with a specialisation in plant pathology and virology. Working for the corporate, national projects, US government international projects on invasive viruses, presenting research in national and international conferences in different countries, and publishing research papers in peer-reviewed international journals for over 25 years, he decided to join Agriculture College in the state of Goa. Taking responsibility as Principal and Dean of Goa College of Agriculture, he strived to get recognition for agricultural education in the state of Goa and is also involved in teaching, projects, and the development of the college campus to provide an environment for the students studying in the four-year professional B.Sc. (Hons.) Agriculture degree programme.

Dr. Kunkalikar has an interest in the traditions and heritage of Goa and participates in seminars and festivals on college campus to share scientific knowledge among people in Goa. Enjoying and drinking the bitter decoction of medicinal plants prepared by his grandmother, he established a medicinal plant garden on the college campus to create awareness of the medicinal use of these plants among students and people.

Carmelito Andrade

Carmelito is a Farmer and Beekeeper from Salcete, Goa. He has keen interest in medical plants and is a big proponent of the same. He also has a Bachelors and Masters Degree in Electronics and Telecommunication engineering and is always advising students/faculty to use open source hardware and software. He has authored multiple books, both technical and non-technical.

Carmelito is a trainer for new upcoming technologies like 3D printing, Internet of Things (IoT) and Edge AI. In addition, he is a certified Drone Pilot and trains students in building and flying custom Drones/Quadcopters.

Carmelito also runs a youtube channel called - DronesGoa which features various Agriculture and Biodiversity videos and Documentaries. In addition, you can also find a playlist on Goan Heritage and various festivals curated by Goencho Festakar, Marius Fernades.

Over the years, inspired by his grandmother's love for agriculture and using medicinal plants for healing, he has collected various medicinal plants, from friends, family and the Forest department of Goa and maintains a small garden of the same.

Acknowledgments

This project would have been impossible without the generous support of our Research team, including Goa's local Healers, Farmers, and Elders. Their contributions form the foundation of this book and provide vital information that allows us to study the healing nature of Medicinal plants in Goa.

The scientific information on Medicinal plants provided by Prof Digambar Mokat is immense value and we profusely thank him.

The support and wisdom by Dr Gwendolyn de Ornelas and Festakar Marius Fernandes, who actually initiated the process of collective decision on collecting traditional knowledge on healing wonders of Medicinal plants in the State of Goa, is highly appreciated.

In addition, we owe a thank you to J Santan Rodrigues (Chairman – Curtorim Biodiversity Management Committe) and Jose Roque Andrade (Chairman – Nuvem Biodiversity Management Committee) for permitting us to take pictures of Medicinal plants in their respective properties and neighbourhood.

Who is this book for?

Goa, beyond the pristine beaches, picturesque landscape and its old indo-portuguese heritage, is also a home to a variety of healing plants and herbs. Indeed, it is the pride of every Goan to boast about its State wealth. These medicinal plants and herbs have been cherished by indigenous communities and traditional healers for their medicinal properties.

The purpose of this book is to explore the rich biodiversity of medicinal plants and their contribution to natural healing. Our intention is to keep the language simple with a little bit of scientific jargon, so that young students can understand and it is simple to follow.

A few of these plants are used on a regular basis like ginger, garlic, coconut and tumeric in preparing our favorite recipes. Neem is used in various soaps and organic pesticides. Many of these were used by our grandparents as remedies to treat cold, fever, skin problems, gastro-interstinal ailments and more.

Also, it is to be noted that most of this information was collected based on our conversation with local Healers and Elders, with some of this confirmed by the Ayurvedic and Scientific community. Some medicinal properties are yet to be confirmed by Researchers/Scientists.

Most of these plants and their tonics have to be taken in moderation, please consult an expert or your elders.

How did this book come about?

The impetus for this book emerged from a seminar held at the Goa College of Agriculture, Old Goa, where Festacar Marius Fernandes, Dr. Gwendolyn de Ornelas and Dr. Digambar Mokat of Savitribai Phule Pune University proposed a collaborative study on the medicinal flora of the region. Organised under the leadership of Dean Dr. Suresh Kunkalikar, the seminar brought together experts and stakeholders and students of various colleges to the study of local plant-based knowledge systems. Mr. Fernandes, serving as Chief Guest, underscored the importance of linking cultural heritage with scientific documentation—a vision that informed the direction of this work.

Following this event, Dean Dr. Suresh Kunkalikar and Carmelito Andrade were entrusted with developing this volume, with contributions and guidance from Dr. Digambar Mokat and inputs from Mr. Fernandes. The idea was to take a multi-disciplinary approach combining field surveys, traditional knowledge and botanical classification. Our methodology involved consultation with local practitioners, examination of existing academic literature and taxonomic identification based on standard botanical references.

1. Aloe Vera

Scientific name: *Aloe Barbadensis miller*
In English: Aloe
Konkani: Katekuor

Aloe vera can be found in most Goan gardens growing in a pot or directly on the ground. It is a cactus-like plant with a short stem and shallow root system. The leaves are fleshy with thorny prickles on the margins, and the flowers are yellow and orange in color. It is also farmed on a large scale in some states of India for cosmetic industry for creams and gels.

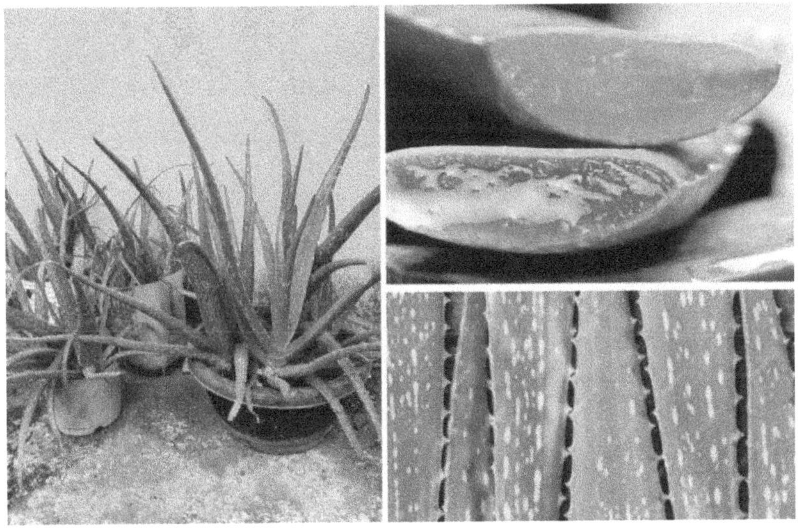

What is used – Leaf Juice, which is a gel-like substance.

Propagation - the most reliable method for propagation is through suckers, which are smaller plants growing alongside the parent plant. It can also be propagated using leaf cuttings, but the suckers method is easier and more successful.

Medicinal benefits

Acne

Pimples form when oil, dead skin cells, and bacteria clog up hair follicles, which then get inflamed and form small bumps, with pus inside. Aloe Vera gel when applied has anti-bacterial and anti-inflammatory properties that help in reducing acne.

Burns

Aloe Vera anti-bacterial and anti-inflammatory effects make it useful for treating burns. Applying a layer of Aloe Vera gel to minor burns and sunburned skin helps the skin heal faster, and reduce redness, itching, and pain. Aloe Vera also helps prevent burns from getting infected.

Aloe Vera gel feels soothing on sunburned skin. It also moisturizes while it heals, which may prevent you from peeling as much.

Constipation

Aloe Vera juice and aloe latex are promoted as a treatment for constipation. Aloe Vera contains substances (such as barbaloin) that act as laxatives. The juice increases the amount of water in the intestine, which makes poop easier to pass and helps digested foods move more easily through the intestines.

Wounds

Slicing the leaf into half and placing it on a wound, helps to prevent infection. And the same method can be used to get rid of impurities from an infected wound.

Jaundice

Use a few drops of Aloe Vera juice in the nostrils to control jaundice.

As a Cosmetic, Aloe Vera is one of the best-known moisturisers and is used in creams and shampoos to retain moisture in skin.

2. Arjun

Scientific name: *Terminalia arjuna*
In English: Arjun tree
Konkani: Arjun

Arjun tree is widely grown in India, and in most parts of Goa. It grows to a height of about 20 meters mostly near rivers, and other water bodies. It grows almost in all types of soils, but prefers humid, fertile loam and red lateritic soils. The tree can also tolerate half submergence for a few weeks, which is ideal for Goa's rainy season. The tree is known for the medical value of its bark. The bark decoction is used in Goa for treating pain, hypertension and heart ailments.

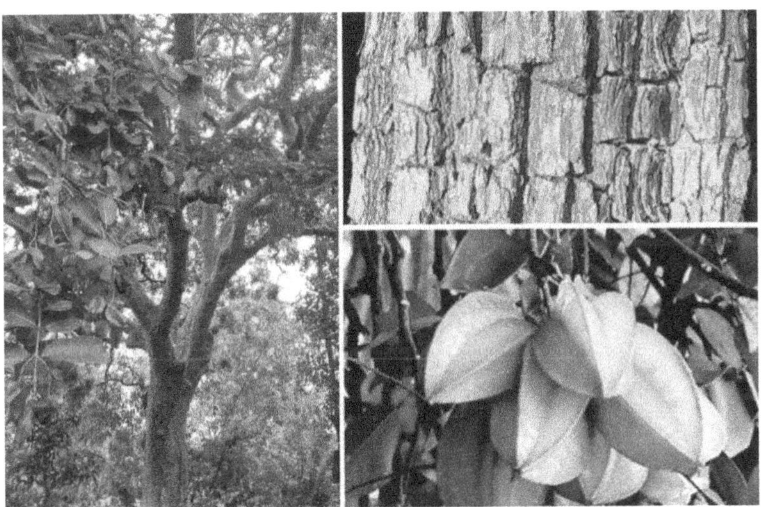

What is used - Bark of the tree

Propagation - The tree is propagated from seeds. First, collect mature fruits from the tree, ensure they are fully ripened, remove the outer husk to access the seeds inside. Later, soak the seeds in water for 24 hours to enhance germination and sow directly in soil.

Medicinal benefits

Wounds and Cuts

To heal wounds, make a decoction of the bark powder and wash wounds with it. This helps with the healing process and speeds up the normalisation of skin.

Fractures

Take a teaspoon of the bark powder every day to facilitate the quick healing of bone tissues at the time of fractures.

Diabetes

Taking a decoction of bark every day is useful in diabetes and regulating blood sugar.

Heart Health

Arjun bark powder is beneficial in managing heart diseases as it acts as a cardiotonic and strengthens the heart muscles. Add two tablespoons of Arjun bark powder to a glass of milk, with four glasses of water and boil it till you get one glass. Take the dose twice a day to keep your heart fit and avoid problems like cholesterol and high blood pressure.

Urinary Tract Infection (UTI)

Arjun tree bark has anti-bacterial properties and taken in powder form can help in management of UTI. Take six tablespoons of Arjun bark powder in a small cup of milk or water, and take it twice a day after lunch and dinner to reduce the symptoms of UTI.

In some cases, the bark powder can be also used as a cosmetic. A face pack of the bark powder and milk can be used every day to lighten dark spots and patches. Caution - it is generally advised to stop consumption of bark powder during pregnancy and also during breastfeeding.

3. Ash Gourd

Scientific name: *Benincasa hispida Cogn*
In English: Ash Gourd
Konkani: Kuvala

Ash Gourd, also known as winter melon, is a vine. When ripe, it has a powdery, ash-colored coating on the surface, which gives it, its name. It's widely consumed in Goa and is often cubed to make a vegetable. Ash Gourd is a good source of vitamins and minerals, including Vitamin C, B-complex, potassium and iron. It is also known for its potential cooling effects.

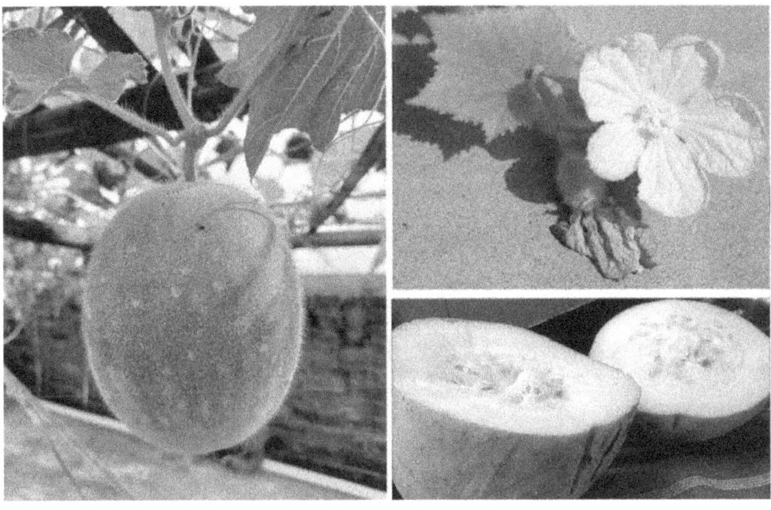

What is used - fruit

Propagation

Ash Gourd is typically propagated by sowing seeds. Seeds are soaked in water for a short period, and then sown in soil beds or containers. After germination, only healthy seedlings are retained for growth.

Medicinal benefits

Boost Immunity

Ash Gourd contains Vitamin C, which is important for white blood cell production. It is also high in zinc, which is another vital element for the immune system.

Digestive Health

Ash Gourd is high in fibre, which promotes healthy gut bacteria, potentially reducing constipation, bloating, and stomach cramps. It also soothes the stomach lining and reduces acidity.

Weight Management

Ash Gourd has a low calorie count and high-water content making it a good choice for hydration and weight management.

Improves skin health

The anti-oxidants and vitamins in Ash Gourd juice contribute to glowing skin, by combating free radicals, reducing wrinkles, and improving texture of skin.

It is also believed that Ash Gourd juice can have a cooling effect on the brain, potentially improving focus and reducing anxiety.

4. Bael

Scientific name: *Aegle marmelos*
In English: Bael
Konkani: Bel

Bael is a 6-12 meters' tall tree, with trifoliate leaves (three leaflets), sharp thorns, and aromatic fruits. Its flowers are greyish white in color, with a sweet scent. The fruit is large and globe-like with many seeds. The fruit is used in various ayurvedic preparations and for its medicinal properties.

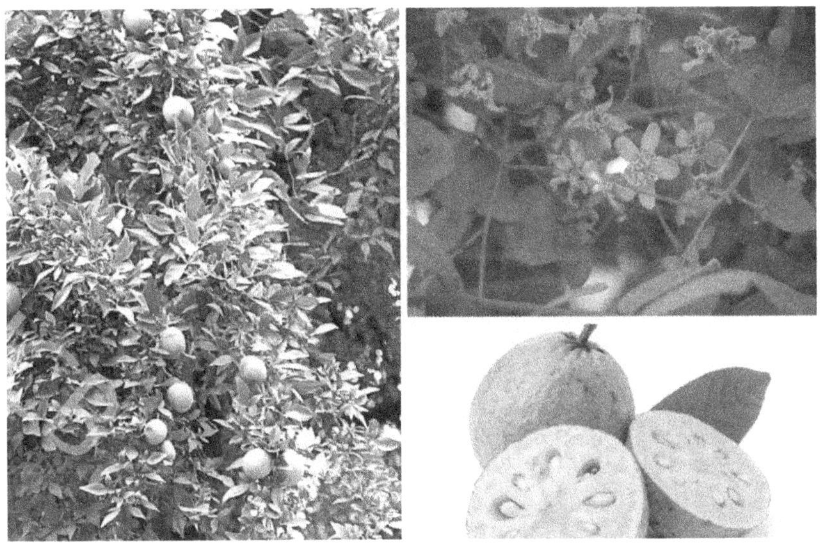

What is used – fruit and leaves

Propagation

Can be propagated both through seeds and grafting. Seed propagation is the traditional method and is sowed typically in June or July. Seedling development is slow, requiring at least a year in the nursery before transplanting.

Medicinal benefits

Diarrhoea

Bael has anti-diarrhoeal and anti-microbial activity. Bael reduces the growth and inhibits the release of toxins by harmful micro-organisms. Bael controls the infection and reduces the frequency of stools in case of diarrhoea. Take half a teaspoon of Bael, churn and mix with water and take after lunch and dinner.

Constipation

Bael might be beneficial in managing constipation. Bael fruit has laxative properties. The ripe fruit of Bael is rich in fibre that helps cleanse the intestine. Have a Bael tea, made of hot water and roasted Bael pulp.

Lowers blood sugar

Bael may lower the blood sugar level. It is generally advised to monitor blood sugar level while taking Bael with other anti-diabetic drugs.

Cosmetic value

Bael pulp can be used as a scrub, basically one to two teaspoons of Bael pulp can be used to gently massage face and neck for 5 to 6 minutes.

Also, it can be used as a Hair pack with coconut oil, which is normally left on hair for 4 to 5 hours and then rinsed with shampoo and water.

5. Banana

Scientific name: *Musa acuminata*
In English: Banana
Konkani: Kellae

Banana is one of the most common fruits in Goa, which needs no introduction as it is consumed by every Goan on a weekly if not daily basis. Most Goan homes have a small area in their backyard where local varieties of bananas are grown. They are soft, sweet, and a good source of some important nutrients.

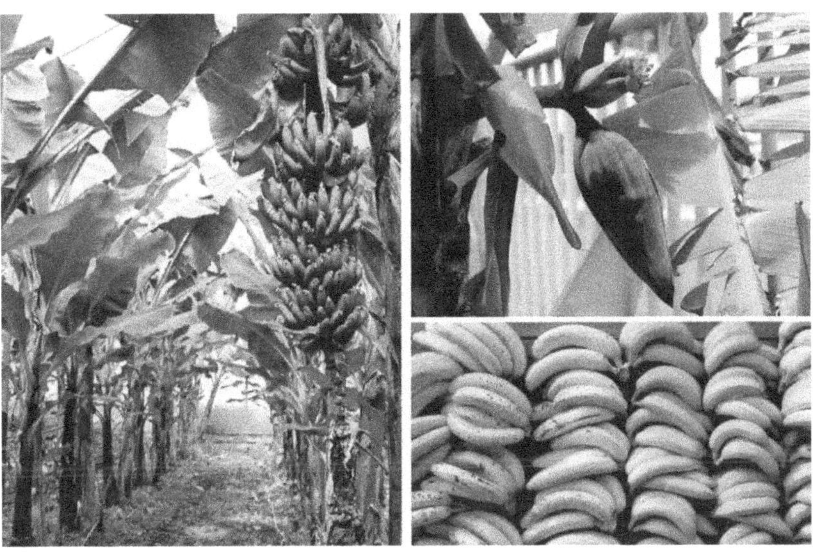

What is used - fruit

Propagation

Banana plants are typically propagated asexually, meaning new plants are grown from parts of the existing plant rather than from seeds. The most common method is through suckers, which are shoots that develop from the underground rhizome at the side of the mother plant.

Medicinal benefits

Digestive health

Banana contains fibre, which helps in digestion. They are good for stomach as they have probiotics, which are the good bacteria found in the gut, and prebiotics, which are carbs that feed on the good bacteria. This plays an important part in controlling how quickly carbohydrates are digested

Green/unripe bananas are a good source of starch, which is a type of carbohydrate that is not digested in small intestine. But it ferments in the large intestine and feeds good bacteria in the gut. Resistant starch can make person feel fuller, which also helps in weight loss. It is also good for constipation.

Faster workout recovery

Bananas can also help with bounce back from strenuous workouts in the gym or strenuous work in field.

Good for Skin

Bananas are rich in manganese, which is good for skin health. It helps with boosting collagen production and makes skin cells more resilient to damage.

Helps with Weight Loss

If a person is on a weight loss diet, bananas can help. With a calorie level of just 100, bananas are nutritious and filling. The fibre and resistant starch also keeps you full for a longer duration, this directly means reducing the quantity of the other high calorie food a person may consume. A medium size banana gives about a quarter of the vitamin B6 needed each day. It helps with metabolism, and plays an important role in helping for better sleep.

Bananas are versatile as well as tasty. They can be eaten ripe, mixed into favourite smoothie/fruit drink, fruit salad, banana bread, or muffins. In the raw form they can be used for various vegetable recipes.

6. Betel Leaves

Scientific name: *Piper betle*
In English: Betel leaves
Konkani: Paan

Betel leaf is a vine, it is a glossy green leaf with a heart shape. It is a common addition to many goan homes and social occasions and family functions, because of its distinct flavour. Beyond its cultural importance, betel leaves have numerous health advantages. These leaves help with digestion, refresh breath, and even have anti-bacterial qualities. They are also rich in anti-oxidants and essential oils.

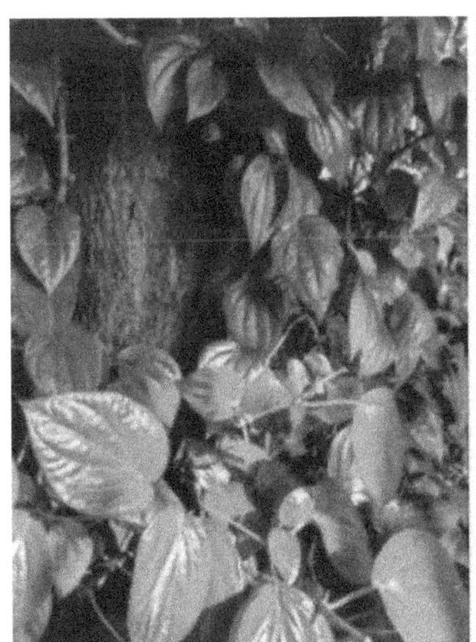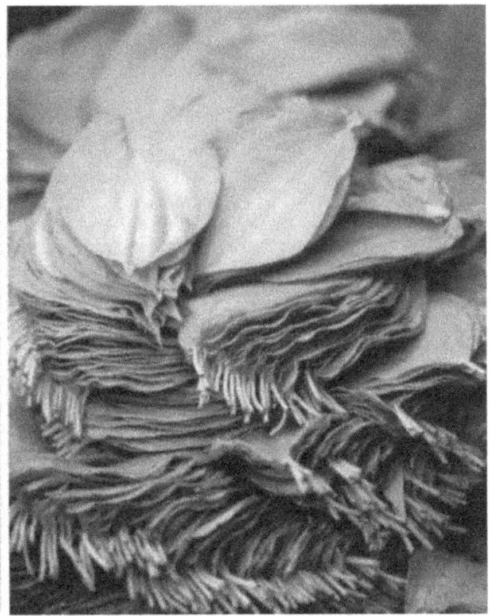

What is used - leaves

Propagation - The betel leaf plant can be propagated by stem cutting. Take a vine of 5 to 6-inch cutting from the main plant and remove the lowermost leaves and place it in moist soil for rooting.

Medicinal benefits

Improve Digestion

After a good meal, betel leaves are consumed, mostly in the inland regions of Goa. The leaf has compounds that help in protecting the gut. Betel leaves increase metabolism triggering circulation and stimulating the intestines to absorb vital vitamins and nutrients.

Anti-fungal properties on infected wounds

Betel leaves have amazing antiseptic properties and compounds that provide protection against germs. It has amazing anti-fungal properties that provide instant relief from fungal infections. Applying the paste of betel leaves kills fungal infection in the affected region.

Improves Oral Health

Betel leaves have numerous anti-microbial agents that effectively combat a host of bacteria in the mouth which trigger bad breath and also helps with issues of cavities. Chewing a tiny amount of leaves paste after meals not only boosts gut wellness but also fights bad breath, as well as relieves toothaches, gum pain and other infections.

Fights Depression

Betel leaves have been used as a natural remedy for stimulating the central nervous system function. The presence of aromatic compounds in betel leaves stimulates the release of compounds, which enhances the sense of well-being and in turn uplifts mood. Chewing betel leaves alone is a simple way to beat depression.

Betel leaves when consumed with tobacco and betel nuts increase the risk of oral cancer. However, it should be noted that betel leaf alone is packed with valuable compounds that have cancer-fighting benefits.

7. Betel Nut

Scientific name: *Areca catechu*
In English: Betel Nut
Konkani: Maadi/Supari

Betel nut is the nut that comes from a plant called Areca. It is pungent, bitter, spicy, sweet, salty, and astringent. It is used to make medicine. Betel nut is chewed alone or in a mixture of tobacco, powdered or sliced betel nut, and other ingredients, just as a caution this is bad for health.

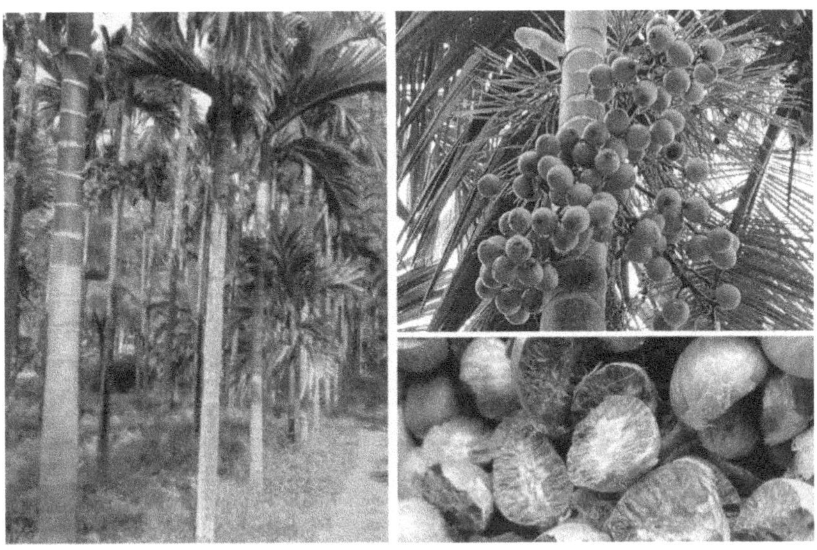

What is used - seed

Propagation

Betel Nut is propagated only by seeds. There are four steps in selection and raising of Betel Nut seedlings, that is - selection of mother palms, selection of seed nuts, germination of seed, raising the seedlings in grow bags and finally selection of seedlings to plant. Each plant should be planted at a distance of 4 meters from each other.

Medicinal benefits

Improves Oral health

Chewing betel nut, especially with betel leaf, is believed to freshen breath and may have anti-bacterial properties that could help prevent cavities.

Used as a Stimulant

Betel nut contains alkaloids, like arecoline, which act as stimulants, potentially leading to increased alertness, reduces fatigue and a mild sense of euphoria.

Helps with Digestion

Chewing the nut stimulates the flow of saliva to aid digestion. Betel nuts also have been used to stimulate the appetite.

Some traditional uses include relieving pain, promoting circulation, and even aiding in weight loss

Chewing betel nuts can make your mouth, lips, and stool turn red. Chewing betel nut regularly throughout the day increases the risk of multiple forms of cancer and cardiovascular disease, with or without added tobacco. Women who chew betel nut formulations, such as paan, during pregnancy significantly increase adverse outcomes for the baby.

8. Bitter Gourd

Scientific name: *Momordica charantia*
In English: Bitter Gourd
Konkani: Karela

Bitter Gourd is commonly eaten as a vegetable in most Goan households. It is widely known for its bitter taste. While preparing a vegetable, the fruit is used after par boiling or soaking in salt water to reduce bitterness. The fruit is a source of several key nutrients. The plant, as a whole contains more than 60 phyto-medicines that are active against more than 30 diseases, including cancer and diabetes. The plant is a slender climbing vine, which is almost 2 to 4 m in height.

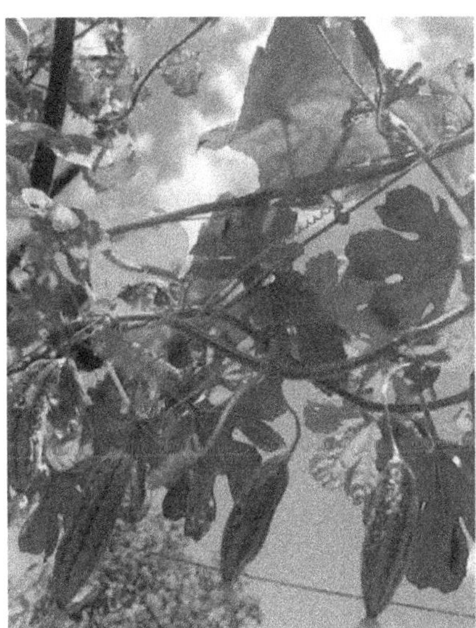 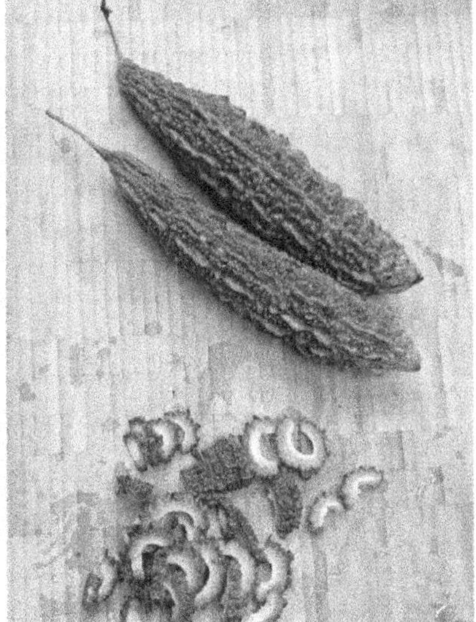

What is used - fruit

Propagation - Bitter gourd can be propagated through seeds by directly sowing them in the soil. Seeds should be sown about half inch deep in good-draining soil, ideally enriched with compost. Providing support like a trellis or wire mesh is essential for the climbing vine as the plant grows.

Medicinal benefits

Managing Diabetes

The bioactive compounds are responsible for the vegetable's bitter taste, but they play a major role in lowering blood sugar levels in people with diabetes. These compounds help move glucose from the blood to the cells while also helping liver and muscles for better process and store glucose. Bitter Gourd can be sliced and boiled for about 10 minutes on a high flame, and given to a diabetic patient.

Fights inflammation

Bitter gourd is packed with compounds, which have the ability to lower inflammation in the body.

Reduce Cholesterol levels

High levels of cholesterol can cause fatty plaque to build up in arteries, forcing heart to work harder to pump blood and increasing risk of heart disease. Consuming bitter gourd as a vegetable or just boiled in water can significantly decrease the levels of LDL (bad cholesterol).

Weight Loss

Bitter gourd is an excellent source of fibre, which is ideal if a person is on a weight loss diet. Fibre passes through your digestive tract very slowly, helping keep one fuller for longer and reducing hunger and appetite. It also has laxative properties, which may help to support digestion and reduce constipation.

Bitter Gourd is difficult to enjoy raw, but has to be cooked in the form of a vegetable. Since it is bitter, it can be mixed with other fruits and vegetables to create a smoothie, making it easy to consume.

9. Black Pepper

Scientific name: *Piper nigrum*
In English: Black Pepper
Konkani: Miri

Black pepper is one of the most commonly used spices worldwide. It has a mild spicy flavor that goes well with many dishes. It is called a "King of spices", and has been used in ancient Ayurvedic medicine for thousands of years. Historically, Black pepper has always been in high demand. It was traded along ancient routes linking India with Egypt and Rome. So much so, that at one time it was used as a form of currency.

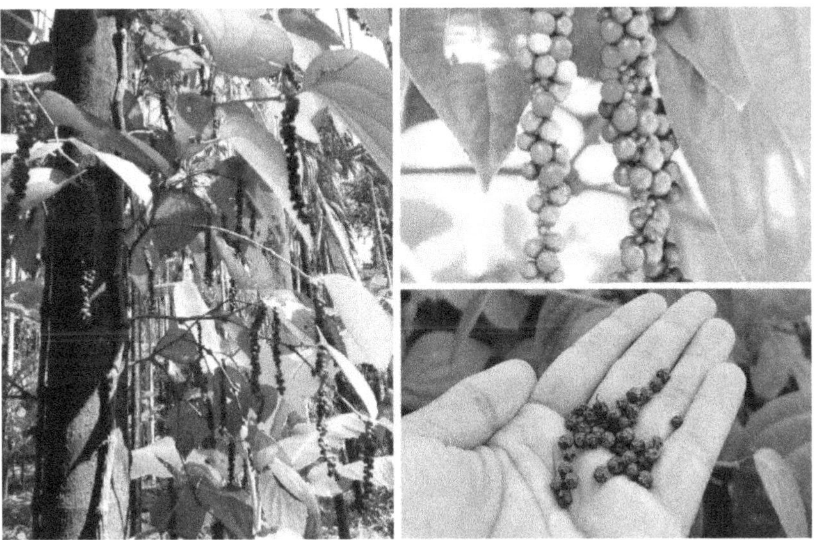

What is used - seed with the dried fruit.

Propagation - Black pepper can be propagated by three main methods: dry seeds, cuttings, or stolons. Cuttings are the most common method for commercial production. They are typically taken from the secondary runners of the plant containing one or two leaves. The rooted black pepper cuttings are planted in polythene bags holding a potting mixture or directly planted on the ground with rich soil, which serves as the mother plant.

Medicinal benefits

Helps with Weight Loss

Black pepper is known to help in weight loss because of its ability to enhance metabolism and reduce fat accumulation. It promotes the breakdown of fat and prevents the accumulation of new fat cells, which makes it an effective natural remedy for obesity.

Black pepper stimulates the production of digestive enzymes, which aid in the digestion of proteins and fats. It helps to reduce bloating and gas, making it a valuable spice for maintaining digestive health. It also stimulates saliva production in the mouth, which is the first step in the digestive process.

Black pepper is rich in anti-oxidants, which promote healthy aging by protecting cells from damage.

Anti-ageing

The anti-oxidants in Black pepper can help to prevent signs of ageing by protecting the skin from damage. Consuming some black pepper reduces the appearance of wrinkles, fine lines and age spots. Black pepper also improves circulation, which can give the skin a healthy glow.

Blood sugar control

Consuming some Black pepper has a positive effect on controlling blood sugar levels and insulin spikes. Also, Black pepper has demonstrated cholesterol-lowering effects.

Beyond its health benefits, black pepper plays an essential role in numerous recipes and culinary applications around the world. From being used as seasoning, to baking and pickling.

Consuming pepper should be in moderation, and overdoing it may lead to the feeling of heartburn or indigestion.

10. Cathedral bells

Scientific name: *Kalanchoe pinnata*
In English: Cathedral Bells
Konkani: Panfuti

Cathedral bells is a distinct plant - the leaves are thick, fleshy, elliptical in shape, and curved, with a serrated margin. The leaves are remarkable for their ability to produce bulbils. When the plantlets fall to the ground, they root and grow to bigger plants. With a growth potential of up to 8 meters, these plants are impressive in stature and bloom with bell-shaped flowers, which make it an ideal plant to enhance the beauty of the garden.

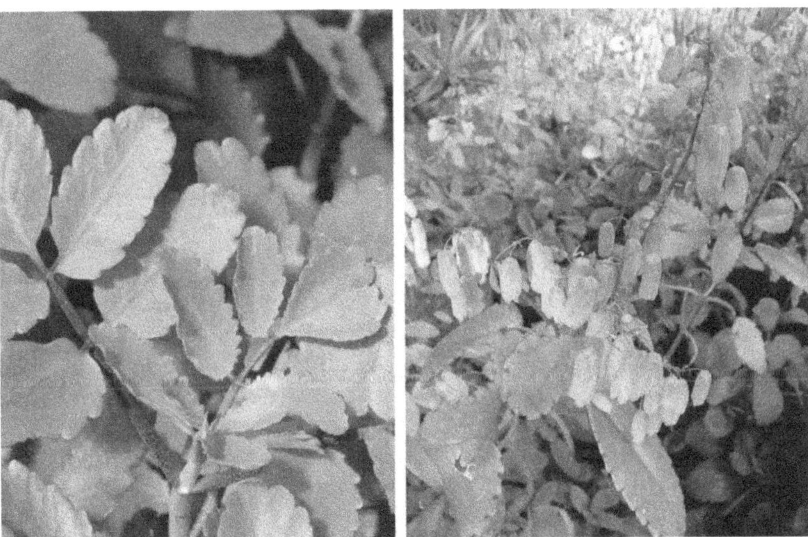

What is used - Leaves

Propagation - Cathedral bells can be propagated using both stem cuttings and leaf cuttings. Stem cuttings are taken from a healthy stem and can be rooted in water or soil. Healthy leaves can be placed in moist soil to develop plantlets along the leaf edges.

Medicinal benefits

Wound Healing

Crushed leaves or leaf juice is applied to wounds to stop bleeding and promote fast healing.

Dissolve Kidney Stones

The plant is used to help dissolve and expel kidney stones.

Treating various skin conditions

Juice made out of the leaves is used for treating boils, ulcers and other skin disorders.

Digestive Issues

Used for treating stomach pain and ulcers.

Respiratory Problems

Herbal tea made from the leaves is used to treat coughs and colds.

Control blood sugar

The plant has been used traditionally to help manage diabetes, by making a decoction of the leaves.

Treating Infections

The plant possesses anti-bacterial, anti-fungal, and anti-viral properties, making it useful for treating infections.

11. Chaff-flower

Scientific name: *Calotropis gigantea*
In English: Chaff flower
Konkani: Aagodo, Rui

Chaff flower is a large shrub that grows about 4 m tall and can be found in the wild as well as urban areas and at the side of buildings/roads in Goa. It has clusters of waxy flowers that are either white or lavender in colour. Each flower consists of five pointed petals and a small crown rising from the center.

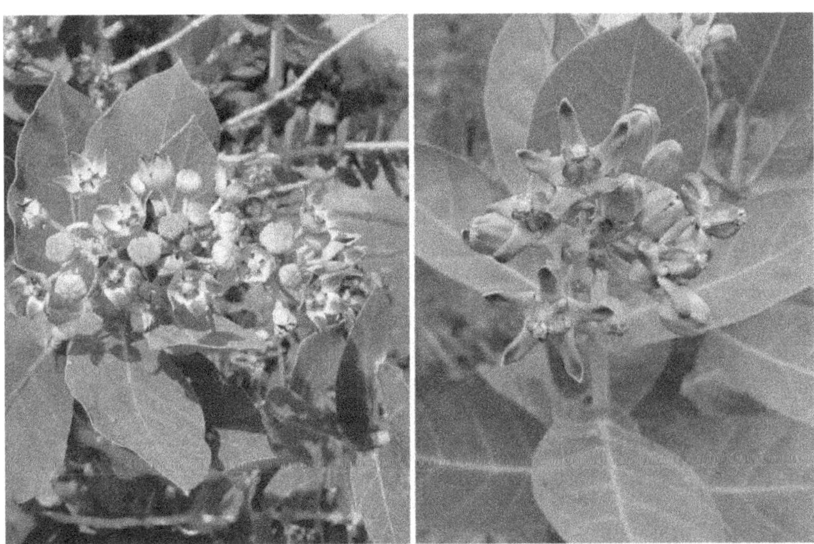

What is used - leaves

Propagation - Chaff flower plant is propagated by seeds or stem cutting. The seeds are spread by water, wind in the wild and are generally pollinated by wasps, bees and butterflies. For planting, sow the seeds in soil and lightly press them into the mix. Keep the soil consistently moist but not waterlogged by misting regularly or using a watering can.

Medicinal benefits

Wound Healing

The latex from the plant contains tannins, which has anti-microbial properties, promoting wound healing and potentially preventing infection.

Reduce Inflammation and joint pain

Take a handful of leaves and boil them for ten minutes. Let it cool and make a fine paste. This leaf paste can be applied over the area of inflammation.

Skin and Digestive Disorders

Chaff flower plant has been used to address skin ailments, digestive issues and even neurological problems.

Respiratory and Circulatory Issues

Chaff flower plant is beneficial for respiratory and circulatory disorders, as well as conditions like fevers and elephantiasis.

In traditional medicine, different parts of the plant, including roots, root bark, flowers, leaves, and juice, have been used in various medicinal formulations.

12. Chaulmoogra Tree

Scientific name: *Hydnocarpus wightianus Blume.*
In English: Chaulmoogra Tree
Konkani: Khosta

Chaulmoogra Tree is particularly known for the oil extracted from its seeds, which has traditionally been used in Ayurveda and other traditional medicine to treat leprosy and skin diseases. The tree grows up to 10 meters tall, with brownish, fissured bark and pinkish blaze. The flowers are small, white, and found in axillary short cymes or solitary. The fruit is woody, and is a globe like berry.

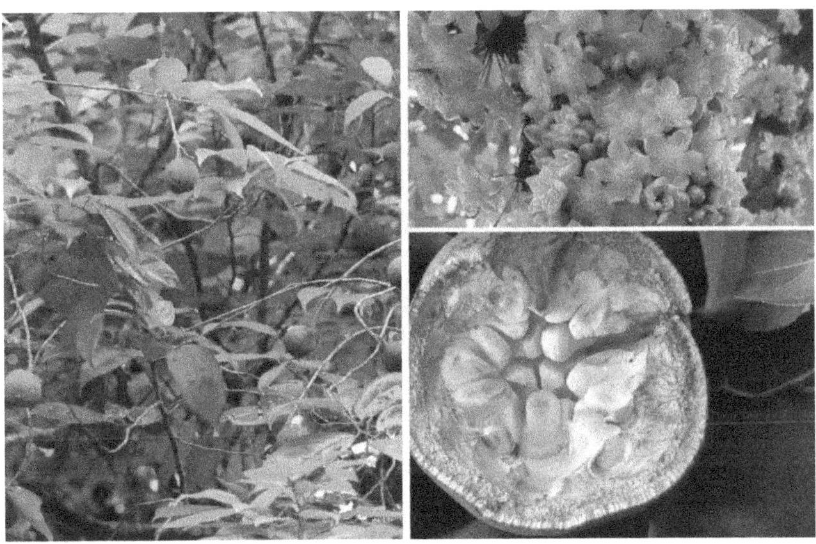

What is used - seed

Propagation

The propagation methods include seed sowing or grafting. The seeds can be collected from ripe fruits, which typically appear in August and September. Sow seeds in drained soil, providing adequate moisture and sunlight. Propagation through grafting is also another option.

Medicinal benefits

Treating Leprosy

Chaulmoogra oil is used for leprosy treatment through topical, oral and even parenteral administration. This oil is extracted by pressing the seeds and is known to heal skin disorders when it is directly applied to affected area on the skin.

Wound Healing

The oil from the seeds can also be used for wound healing as it increases the strength of collagen tissues.

Reducing Fevers

Chaulmoogra has a calming effect, which is helpful in reducing fevers.

Chaulmoogra is unsafe when taken by mouth because it contains cyanide and might cause cyanide poisoning. It can cause cough, difficulty in breathing, throat spasms, kidney damage, head and muscle pain and even paralysis.

13. Chebulic Myrobalan

Scientific name: *Terminalia chebula Retz*
In English: Chebulic Myrobalan
Konkani: Hardo

Chebulic Myrobalan is used for bowel regulation and is used as a gentle laxative. It is also known for its use in beauty and wellness products. The Chebulic Myrobalan tree is celebrated for its numerous health benefits and is also called the King of medicine

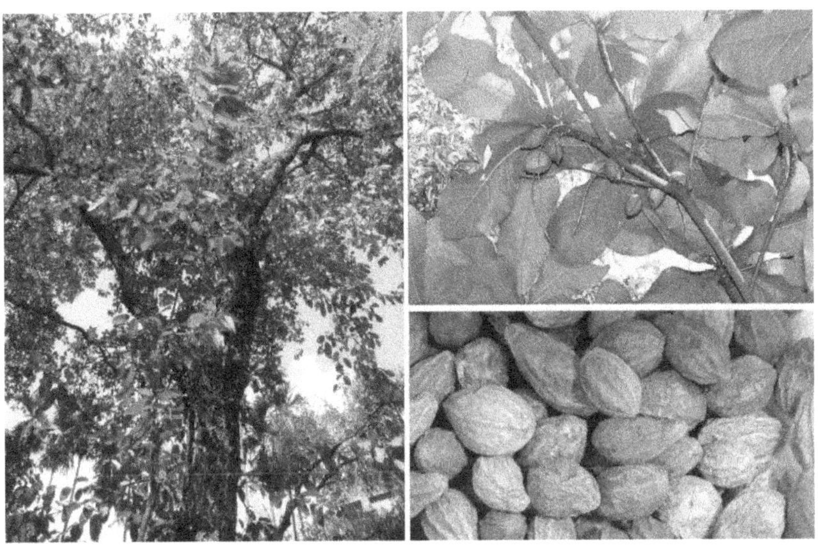

What is used - fruit, leaves

Propagation - Mostly via seeds, but cuttings and grafting methods can also be used in propagation.

Medicinal benefits

Impoves body immunity

The fruit of the Chebulic myrobalan is rich in compounds, which are known for their anti-oxidant effects. These compounds help neutralize free radicals in the body, reducing oxidative stress and lowering the risk of chronic diseases.

The tree has been found to enhance immune function, making it an excellent natural remedy for boosting overall health and resilience against infections.

Digestive health

Traditionally, this has been used as a digestive aid. It can enhance gut health by promoting the growth of beneficial gut bacteria and improving digestion.

Anti-Inflammatory effects

The anti-inflammatory properties of the tree help reduce inflammation in the body, which is linked to numerous health conditions.

Cardiovascular health

It helps to lower cholesterol and improve heart health. It has the ability to reduce oxidative stress and contributes to cardiovascular protection.

Improves skin health

The anti-oxidant properties help combat signs of aging, such as wrinkles and fine lines. It is often used in face masks and creams to promote a youthful appearance. It is effective in treating acne and reducing blemishes. It helps soothe irritated skin and prevent breakouts.

Hair Health

The fruit is also used in hair care products to promote healthy hair growth and prevent dandruff. Its nourishing properties help strengthen hair follicles and improve scalp health.

In addition to its health benefits, the tree plays a crucial role in the environment. It is a hardy tree that can thrive in a variety of soil types and climatic conditions, making it an excellent species for reforestation efforts.

14. Cinnamon

Scientific name: *Cinnamomum verum*
In English: Cinnamon
Konkani: Tiki

Cinnamon, commonly found in most Goan kitchens, is a spice that comes from the dried bark of cinnamon trees. Cinnamon is used mainly as an aromatic property and flavouring additive in a wide variety of vegetable and meat dishes. This includes sweet and savoury dishes, snack foods, teas, hot chocolate and all kinds of traditional foods. Cinnamon is an evergreen tree characterized by oval-shaped leaves, thick bark and a berry fruit. When harvesting the spice, the bark and leaves are the primary parts of the plant used.

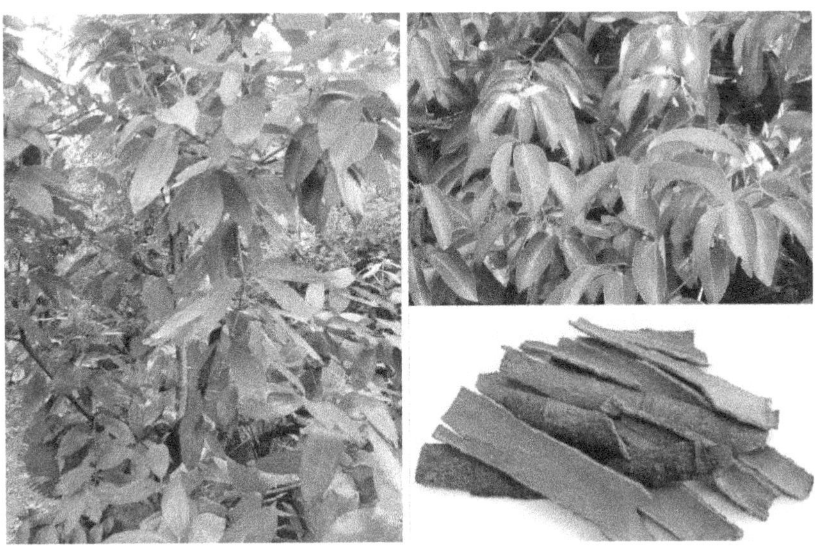

What is used - bark of tree, leaves

Propagation

To grow a cinnamon plant, start with selecting a location with sandy or lateritic soil and adequate rainfall. Plant during the monsoon season (June to August) for optimal establishment. Either seeds, cuttings, or seedlings from a nursery can be used.

Medicinal benefits

Helps with weight loss

Cinnamon helps with weight loss and obesity-related diseases. It increases hormones that help regulate fat metabolism.

Improves memory

Cinnamon improves memory and cognitive function. Its extract helps with Alzheimer's disease.

Helps reduce Diabetes

Cinnamon could be beneficial in managing type 2 diabetes by helping to regulate blood sugar and cholesterol levels.

Anti-Viral

Cinnamon also helps protect against certain viruses, including influenza and mosquito-derived dengue fever.

Increases body Immunity

Like other spices, cinnamon contains plant compounds that have anti-oxidant and anti-inflammatory properties, which help regulate blood pressure. It is good for skin health and helps protect against bacterial and fungal infections.

A traditional use for cinnamon has been as a tooth powder to treat toothache and other dental problems including bacterial overgrowth and bad breath.

15. Cloves

Scientific name: *Syzygium aromaticum*
In English: Cloves
Konkani: Kalaphur

Cloves are the aromatic flower buds of a tree. The clove tree is an evergreen tree that grows up to 8 to 12 meters tall, with large leaves and crimson flowers grouped in clusters. The flower buds initially have a pale hue, gradually turn green and then transition to a bright red which means they are ready for harvest. Cloves are harvested at 1.5 to 2 centimetres long. Cloves can be found in every goan house and are used in various vegetable and meat dishes.

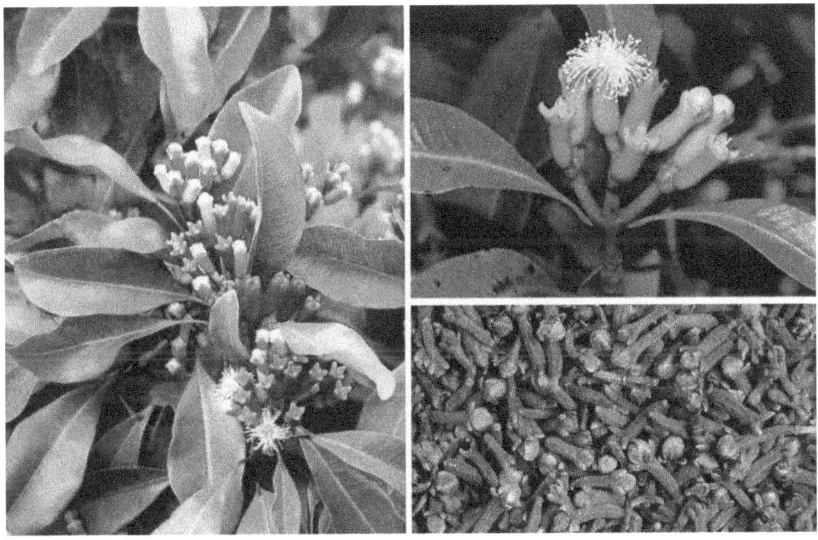

What is used - flower buds

Propagation - Clove is propagated from seeds, which are planted soon after harvest. Seeds should be collected and extracted from the fruits of healthy mother plants. The seeds are extracted by soaking the fruits in water and peeling the skin from the fruit. The seeds are sowed one fourth inch deep.

Medicinal benefits

Relief Toothache

To kill the bacteria causing the toothache, take a piece of clove and place it on the affected tooth, which will give temporary relief. Due to its anti-bacterial properties, cloves can prevent gum infections and reduce bad breath.

Improves Digestion

Cloves stimulate the production of digestive enzymes, which help break down food and improve nutrient absorption. This makes them especially helpful for people dealing with bloating, gas and indigestion. To improve digestion, make a clove tea with ginger and honey, this will help soothe the stomach and help with digestion.

Boost immune system

Cloves are known for its anti-microbial properties, helping fight infections and boosting the body's immune system. Cloves, in addition to being a flavorful rich spice, are rich in essential nutrients such as fiber, vitamins and minerals. Incorporating a couple of ground cloves into your diet can provide a nutritional boost.

Relieves congestion and cough

The warming properties can help relieve symptoms of coughs, colds, and asthma. Clove helps to clear mucus from the airways and makes it easier to breathe. A common solution involves boiling cloves in water and inhaling the steam to relieve congestion. This simple method can provide immediate relief for those suffering from respiratory issues.

The next time you're in the kitchen, consider adding cloves to your dishes for a delicious and healthy boost. Create spice blends using cloves for added flavour and health benefits. A homemade chai (tea) spice mix might include cloves, cinnamon, ginger, and cardamom. This blend can be used to prepare a fragrant and health-boosting tea. By experimenting with cloves in cooking, enjoy their flavour while reaping their many health benefits.

16. Coconut

Scientific name: *Cocos nucifera*
In English: Coconut
Konkani: Maad/Nall

Coconut palms are spotted everywhere in Goa. It is a palm where each and every part of the palm has some kind of use and is called the "tree of life". Coconut's maturity impacts the way it is used and how it is processed. The younger green coconut is typically used for its water and kernel. As the coconut ages, the kernel solidifies and the water content decreases and this is mostly used in vegetables and the famous goan fish curry recipes. The oil is typically extracted from mature coconut.

What is used - nuts

Propagation - Coconut is propagated through seedlings. Choose a coconut, which sloshes the water inside when it is shaken. Soak the coconut in water for two days and place in soil just to cover half coconut with soil. A coconut will germinate in three to four months.

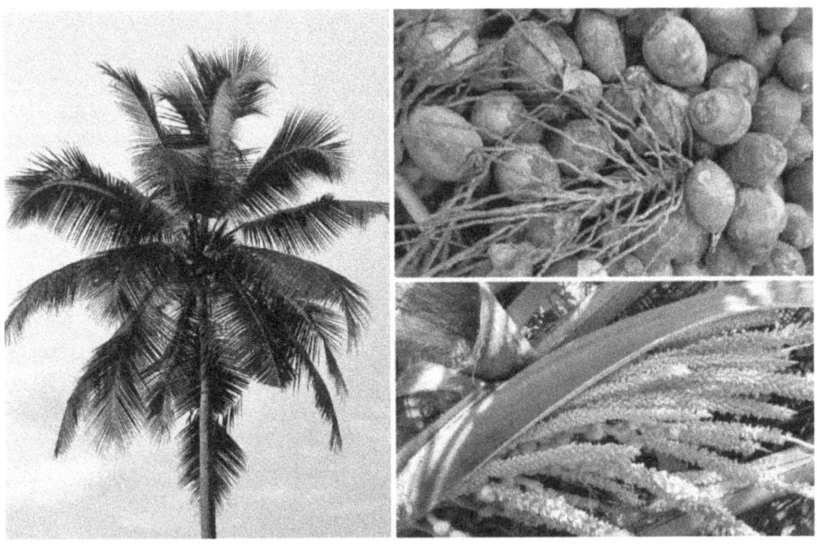

Medicinal benefits

Strengthening the immune system

Coconut contains compounds with anti-oxidant and anti-inflammatory properties. They strengthen the immune system and protect body against infections by fungi, viruses and bacteria.

Weight loss

When consumed in moderate quantities, coconut can help to keep the stomach full between meals. This effect can reduce overall food intake during meals and help in reducing weight.

Regulating blood pressure

Coconut has good amount of potassium, a mineral that helps in elimination of excess sodium from the body. This regulates blood pressure and prevents the risk of cardiac ailments.

Hydration

During summers Coconut is rich in minerals such as potassium and manganese, which makes it a great source for replenishing minerals that are lost through diarrhoea, vomiting and even a gym workout.

Fighting constipation

Coconut is rich in insoluble fibre, which helps with natural bowel movements and adds bulk/hardness to the stool.

In most goan homes, tender coconut water is provided to women during pregnancy, as coconut is known to have a lot of minerals.

17 Cumin

Scientific name: *Cuminum cyminum*
In English: Cumin
Konkani: Jeere

The dried seeds of the Cumin plant are used as a spice especially in vegetable cooking. It is also used as a seasoning for meats. Both cumin seed and powder have a rich, earthy, nutty flavor. Cumin packs a lot of health benefits into a few tiny seeds. The Cumin plant grows to 30–50 cm tall and is mostly harvested by hand.

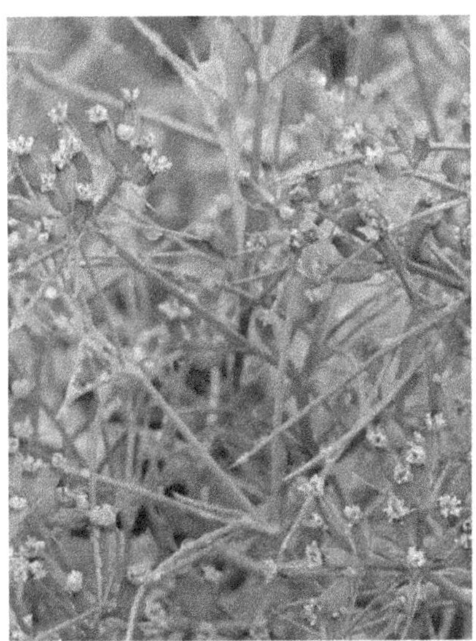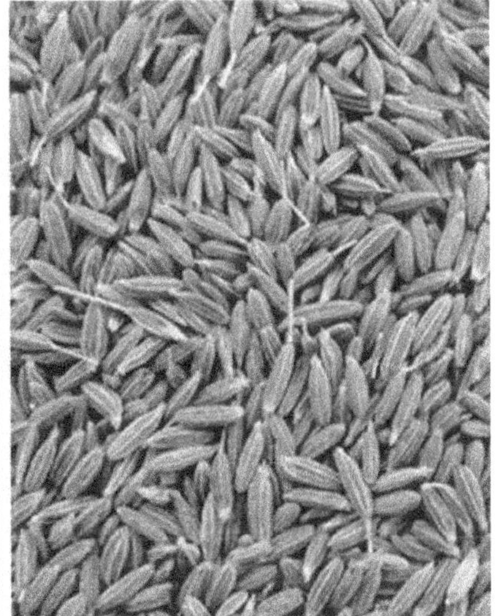

What is used - seed

Propagation

Cumin is primarily propagated through seeds, which are sown in soil. The ideal time for sowing is winter months, specifically November or December, when the climate is moderately warm and cool. Seeds can be sown either by broadcasting or placing in rows, with a spacing of 30 cm between rows.

Medicinal benefits

Improve Digestion

Cumin can help in digestion. The extract or cumin boiled in water for 5 minutes can be consumed to get relief from irritable bowel syndrome symptoms like belly pain and bloating. Cumin has also been a popular remedy for diarrhoea.

Anti-bacterial effects

Cumin seeds help in killing some harmful bacteria in the body. It kills and prevents *E. coli*, a type of bacteria that causes food poisoning.

Controlling Cholesterol

Cumin helps control cholesterol levels. Cumin powder dissolved in yogurt reduces LDL (bad cholesterol) and triglycerides while increasing HDL (good cholesterol).

Weight Loss

Cumin can help in reducing weight when consumed as part of a healthy diet. Cumin powder is known to reduce weight, fat mass, and Body Mass Index (BMI).

Cumin contains compounds, which work as anti-oxidants in the body. Anti-oxidants can help neutralize unstable particles called free radicals that cause cell damage, which in turn can help prevent diseases like cancer, heart disease, and high blood pressure.

18 Custard Apple

Scientific name: *Annona squamosal*
In English: Custard Apple
Konkani: Sitafal

Custard apple is a fruit with a creamy, sweet, and aromatic flesh. The fruit has a hard, thin skin, and the pulp is granular, sweet and encloses a cluster of flesh-covered seeds. The fruit can be eaten fresh by removing the flesh from the hard skin and seeds. It is also used in various desserts, including ice cream, fruit creams, and pastries. The plant is normally a small, well-branched tree/shrub.

What is used - fruit

Propagation

Custard apple seeds germinate in 2-4 weeks with proper soaking and temperature. Trees mature in 3-4 years, yielding multiple fruiting cycles over 15-20 years. Custard apples thrive in warm climates; the ideal temperatures are 20°C to 30°C.

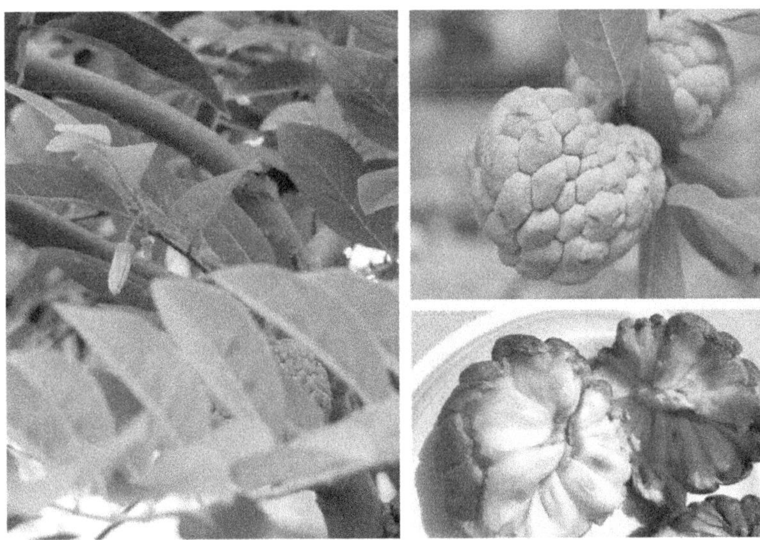

Medicinal benefits

Digestive Health

Custard apples are a good source of fibre, which promotes healthy digestion and prevents constipation.

Immunity Booster

Custard apples provide essential vitamins, minerals, and anti-oxidants, which can help support overall health and protect against cellular damage. Vitamin C, found in many fruits, is a powerful anti-oxidant that can boost the immune system.

Weight Management

Custard apples can be a healthy part of a balanced diet, with some fruits like ambarella being low in calories and high in fibre, promoting satiety and aiding in weight management.

Gut Health

Custard apples like apples contain pectin, a type of fibre that acts as a probiotic, supporting the growth of beneficial gut bacteria.

19. Edible Stemmed Vine

Scientific name: *Cissus quadrangularis*
In English: Edible Stemmed Vine
Konkani: Hadjod

Edible Stemmed Vine is a perennial vine. Traditionally, its parts are dried and made into powder to use as a medicine. It is known to help stimulate bone growth, and a must have for people with fractures, joint pain, low bone mass and many other conditions. It can be consumed as a simple vegetable made with onion and few other spices for taste.

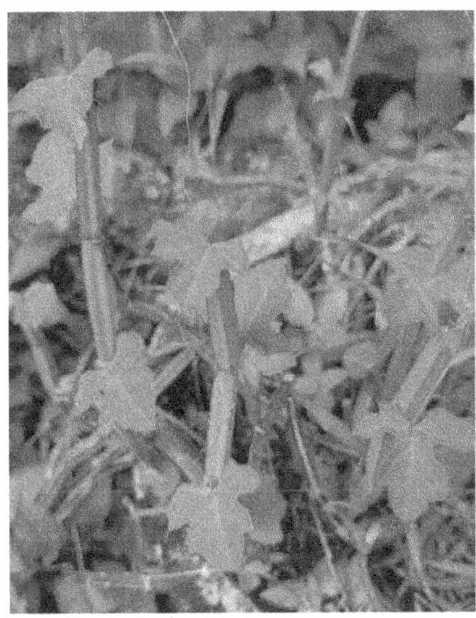
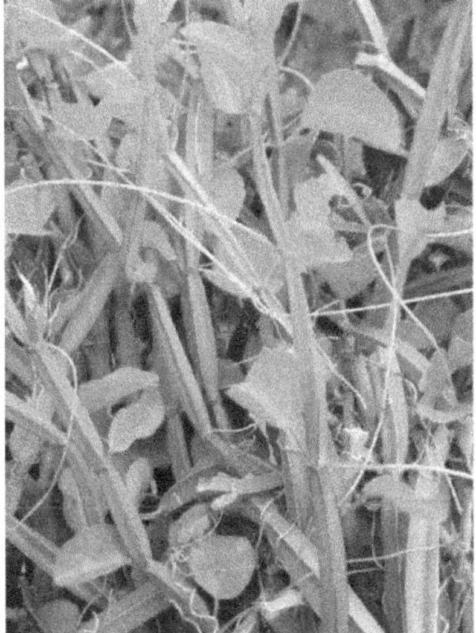

What is used - Stem of the vine

Propagation - Propagate Edible Stemmed Vine through stem cuttings - take cuttings during the growing season, allow them to callous over for a few days and then plant in a well-draining soil or a pot.

Medicinal benefits

Improves Bone Health

Edible Stemmed Vine is known to have anti-inflammatory and bone-strengthening properties. It helps promote bone fracture healing and is also know to help in osteoporosis.

Improves Joint Health

It helps in joint pain and inflammation. Also, it is beneficial for arthritis.

Boost body immunity

It contains compounds with anti-oxidant properties, which prevent the formation of free radical that can cause long term diseases. It has been used traditionally for various other conditions, including diabetes, infections and allergies.

Weight Management

The plant used as a vegetable is known to help in reducing body weight and fat mass. It is known to inhibit enzymes involved in fat storage.

20. Fenugreek

Scientific name: *Trigonella foenum-graecum*
In English: Fenugreek
Konkani: Methi

Fenugreek looks like a clover, with small yellow, white, or purplish-blue flowers and golden-brown seeds inside a pod. Fenugreek seeds are pungent-sweet in smell and taste, making them perfect to add to recipes where a hint of sweetness is needed in vegetable. The seeds and leaves are used in salad and vegetables.

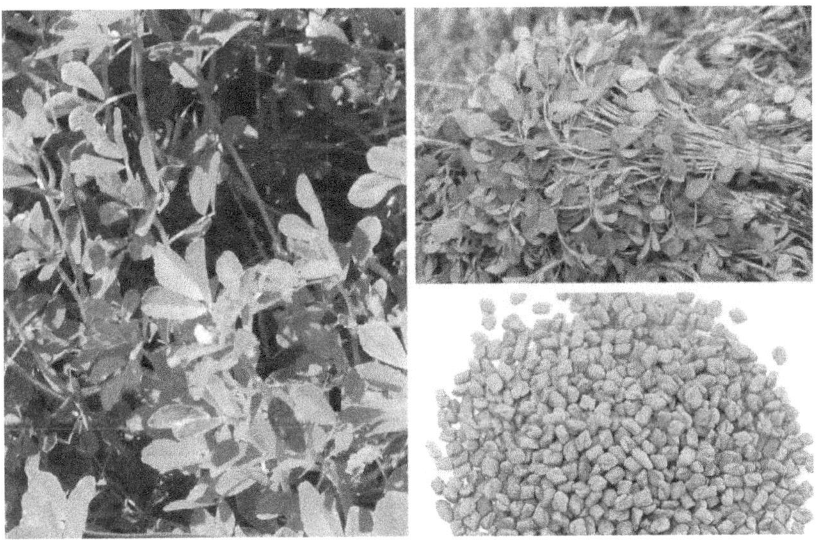

What is used - seed, leaves

Propagation - Fenugreek is propagated from seed. The seed should be directly sown to a depth of 1–2 cm and about 7.5 cm distance between individual plants. It may also be spread by broadcasting by hand.

Medicinal benefits

Digestive Health

Fenugreek is a good source of fibre, which means it can aid digestion and prevent constipation. It has been found to help reduce bloating and gas.

Lactation Support for breastfeeding mothers

Fenugreek is traditionally used to increase breast milk supply in mothers. Breastfeeding mothers who drank/added fenugreek to tea increased their milk production for babies.

Menstrual Cramps in women

Fenugreek helps reduce menstrual cramps and other symptoms associated with menstruation. It also helps alleviate menopause symptoms like hot flashes.

Blood sugar regulation

Fenugreek seeds help lower blood sugar levels in people with diabetes by slowing down sugar absorption in the stomach and stimulating insulin production. Basically, fenugreek can improve insulin sensitivity and reduce blood glucose levels.

21. Flame/Glory Lily

Scientific name: *Glorisa superba*
In English: Flame/Glory Lily
Konkani: Arthi/wag

Glory Lily is found sparsely in between bushes in various parts of Goa. It is easily identified by its unique flowers, which are large on long pedicles with wavy margins, with the upper half, which is crimson red in colour and the base of the flower is bright yellow. The plant is a perennial climbing herb. The plant is known for its potential anti-inflammatory, analgesic and anti-arthritic properties, making it a remedy for conditions like arthritis, rheumatism, inflammation and more.

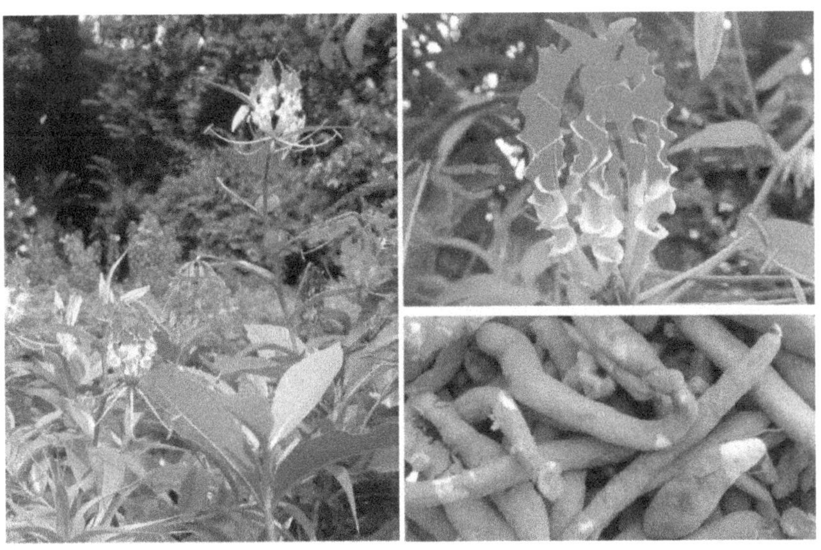

What is used -Underground tubers

Propagation

It can be propagated by seed, but mostly the rhizome is used. Dig up the rhizome in spring after the plant has shed its leaves. Divide the rhizome with a knife and replant it.

Medicinal benefits

Skin Diseases

Glory Lily is used in traditional medicine for treating skin diseases, including leprosy and parasitic skin infections. Tubers are crushed and applied externally in the form of a paste.

Arthritis and Rheumatism

The plant's anti-inflammatory and analgesic properties make it useful for managing arthritis and rheumatism

Treat Digestive issues

It's used to treat indigestion, colic, and piles. Decoction of tubers is used as a tonic, laxative in deworming and abdominal pain.

Reducing Fever

Glory Lily has antipyretic (fever-reducing) properties and is also used to address snakebites.

Glory Lily contains colchicine and other alkaloids, making it highly poisonous if ingested in large quantities. It's crucial to handle this plant with caution and under the guidance of a Healer or Elder.

22. Garlic

Scientific name: *Allium cepa*
In English: Garlic
Konkani: Lasun

Raw white garlic can be found in all goan households, used in the preparation of various vegetables and meats. Chopped and raw, it tastes pungent and sharp. It is a herb with simple long, flat leaves and a white bulb-like rhizome.

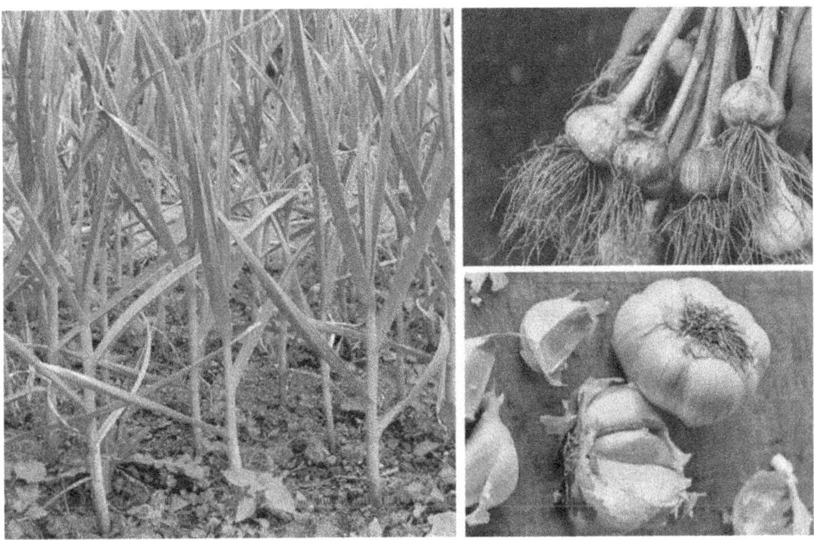

What is used - garlic bulb

Propagation - Garlic does not produce true seed but is propagated by planting cloves, which are the small segments making up the garlic bulb. Each bulb usually contains a dozen or more cloves, each clove is planted separately. Select only larger outer cloves of the best garlic bulbs for planting.

Medicinal benefits

Prevent infections

Garlic is widely recognized for its ability to fight bacteria, viruses, and fungi. It also has anti-viral properties.

Reduce Blood pressure

High blood pressure is one of the root causes of some fatal diseases, like heart attack and stroke. Consuming garlic in its raw form is known to reduce high blood pressure. It reduces the formation of blood clots.

Reduce Cholesterol

Cholesterol is another major reason for heart diseases. Garlic helps lower total LDL (bad cholesterol).

Treating infected wounds

To treat wounds and cuts make a fine paste of garlic and apply on wounds

Improves athletic performance

Older generations used garlic to reduce fatigue and improve the work capacity. In addition, raw garlic juice and its extract have anti-stress properties.

Clears up skin

Garlic's anti-bacterial properties and anti-oxidants can clear up skin by killing acne-causing bacteria. Rubbing raw garlic over pimples can clear the acne.

Treats athlete's foot

Garlic also helps in fighting fungus. Athlete's foot can be soaked in garlic lukewarm water to kill itch-causing fungus

Additionally, garlic is used in food preservation along with salt.

23. Ginger

Scientific name: *Zingiber officinale*
In English: Ginger
Konkani: Aale

Ginger is another plant that needs no introduction as it is commonly used in every household. Ginger has been used in traditional medicine in Goa for centuries. In most Goan households ginger is grown in the backyard. The root rhizomes are dug out from soil when the stalk withers and is washed and scraped, to prevent them from sprouting. Ginger can be used for a variety of recipes such as vegetables, to marinate meats, pickles, and alcoholic beverages.

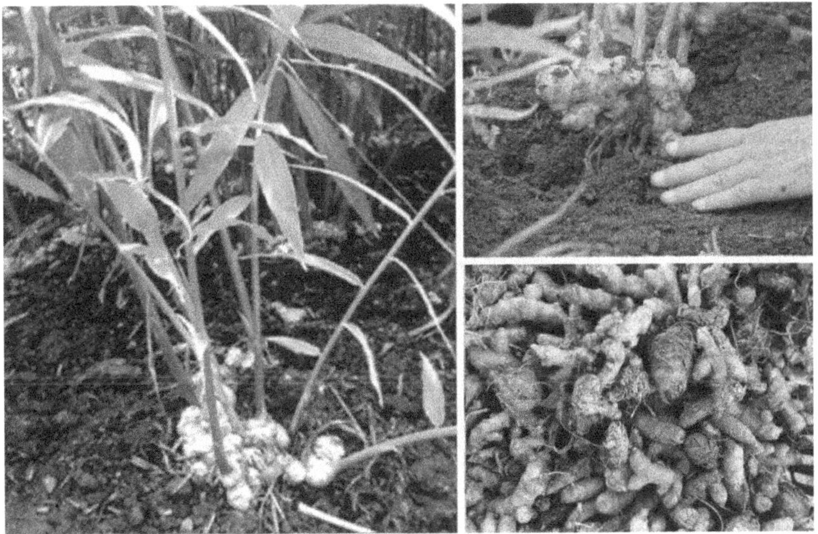

What is used - Ginger rhizome/root

Propagation - Ginger is typically propagated asexually by dividing the rhizome into sections, each containing at least one bud. These sections, called sets, are then planted directly into the soil.

Medicinal benefits

Fighting Germs

Certain chemical compounds 'gingerols' in fresh ginger which helps body ward off germs and is especially good in reducing the growth of bacteria. The bacteria cause mouth infection and affect teeth and in some cases cause serious gum infection.

Ginger is loaded with anti-oxidants, compounds that prevent stress and damage the body. They help the body fight off chronic diseases like high blood pressure, heart disease and promote healthy ageing.

Relief from Sore Throat

One of the common uses of ginger is it has anti-inflammatory and anti-bacterial properties and can be chewed directly or added to a tea to get temporary relief from a sore throat.

Eases Arthritis Symptoms

Ginger is anti-inflammatory, which means it has the property to reduce swelling. That may be especially helpful for treating symptoms of rheumatoid arthritis. A person might get relief from pain and swelling either by consuming ginger or by applying ginger paste on swollen area.

Relieves Indigestion

In chronic indigestion, consuming ginger will bring some relief. Ginger before meals may help in improving digestion. Basically ginger helps increase the way food moves through the gastrointestinal tract, fighting off indigestion.

It also helps reduce nausea, but large doses of ginger can cause gas, heartburn or diarrhoea.

Relieves Pain

Consuming fresh ginger or ginger tea helps in slowly relieving pain caused by menstrual cramps.

In addition to its medical benefits for thousands of years, ginger has been used for cooking and now also added to soda water.

24. Green Chiretta

Scientific name: *Andrographis paniculata*
In English: Green Chiretta
Konkani: Kirayte

The Green Chiretta is a plant known for its bitter taste. It contains compounds, which are effective in preventing viral replication and also has anti-inflammatory qualities. It is often used to treat and relieve common cold and diarrhoea. It can be found growing in the wild or in Goan gardens.

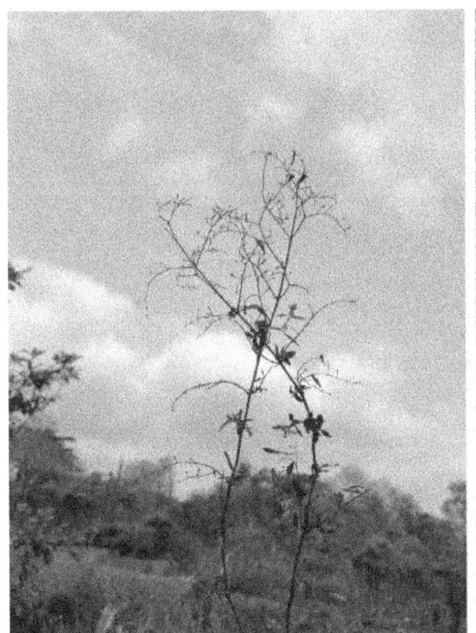
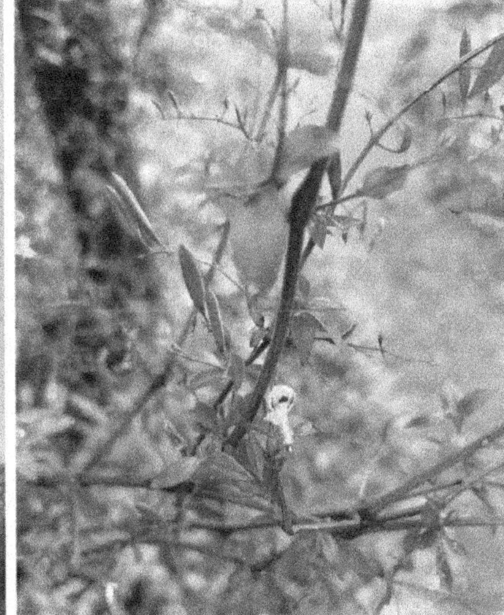

What is used - leaves

Propagation - It is propagated through both seeds and stem cuttings. Seed propagation involves soaking seeds in water for 24 hours, drying them and then sowing in a well-drained, fertile soil mix. Stem cuttings, from one year-old plants, can be planted in moist soil.

Medicinal benefits

Medication for Diabetes

Green Chirata is known to lower blood sugar levels. Boiling the leaves in water and consuming once in two days helps lower blood sugar level in diabetic patients.

Reduce stomach worms

The plant with leaves is dried and stored for use. A decoction is made by boiling leaves and about half a glass is drunk in the morning before breakfast.

Improves liver health

Support liver function and promote detoxification as it helps protect the liver from damage caused by toxins and pollutants, enhancing its ability to metabolise and maintain good health.

Prevents infection on cuts/wounds

A leaf paste can be applied to the skin to treat wounds, cuts and skin infections as it has anti-microbial properties.

Green chiretta supplements are available in various forms, such as capsules and extracts, which are widely used to harness their therapeutic benefits. These supplements are often used to support immune function, promote liver health and alleviate inflammatory conditions.

25 Himalayan wormwood

Scientific name: *Artemisia parviflora L.*
In English: Himalayan wormwood
Konkani: Manpatari

Himalayan wormwood is an aromatic herbaceous perennial with a strong scent. It is used for various digestive problems, such as, loss of appetite, digestion, gallbladder disease and intestinal spasms. It is also helpful for fever, liver disease and muscle pain and worm infection. Though this is commonly found in Himalayan region, it is also found in Goa. It is herbaceous perennials with branching stems and leaves. It possesses a strong, characteristic aroma.

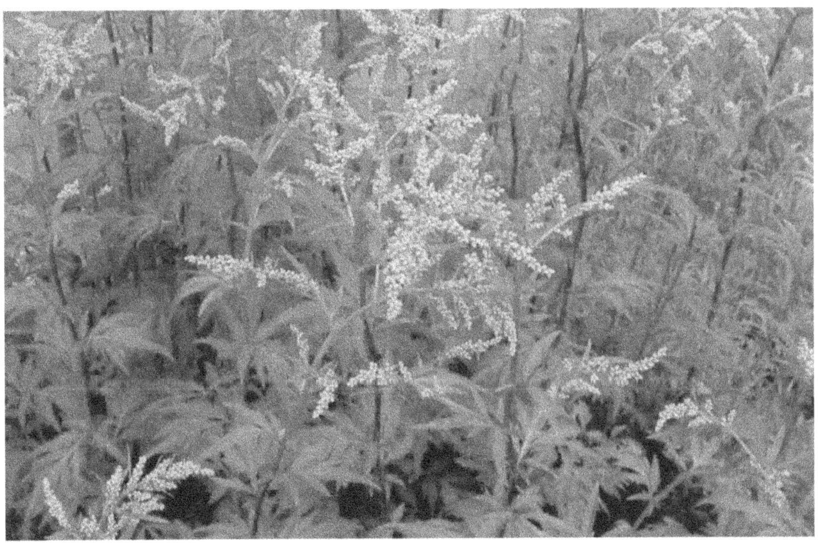

What is used - leaves

Propagation - It can be propagated by seeds or cuttings. Seeds should be sown in soil and lightly covered with soil. The plant cuttings can be used for propagation.

Medicinal benefits

Regulates blood sugar

This herb may hold promise for treatment for type 2 diabetes, since it has been shown to lower blood sugar levels

Hair and Scalp health

Wormwood has anti-bacterial properties, thus inhibiting the growth and activity of bacteria on the scalp. It's extract contains anti-oxidant compounds, such as, flavonoids, polyphenols and tannins, which protect the hair follicles against free radicals.

Alleviate pain

Wormwood has long been sought for its pain-relieving and anti-inflammatory properties. It is mostly used for pain by joint inflammation. Studies suggest that Wormwood may help relieve Crohn's disease, which is characterized by inflammation of lining of the digestive tract.

Wormwood is typically consumed as a decoction or tea.

26 Holy Basil

Scientific name: *Ocimum tenuiflorum*
In English: Holy Basil
Konkani: Tulsi

The Holy Basil is a small annual or short-lived perennial shrub, which can grow up to one meter in height. The fragrant leaves are green or purple, depending on the variety. The Holy Basil plant is revered in Hinduism as a manifestation of the Goddess Lakshmi (Tulsi), the principal consort of the God Vishnu.

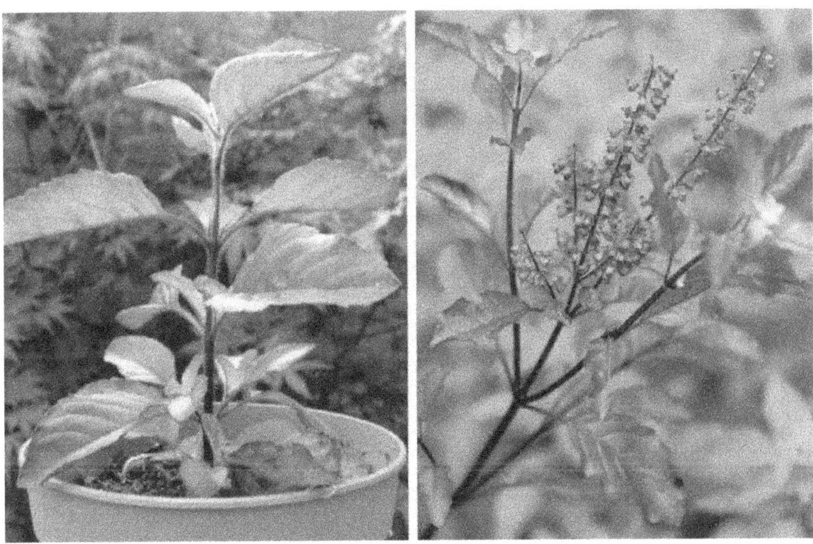

What is used - leaves

Propagation - Cut a six-inch stem just below the leaf node where roots emerge. Plant in soil with a mixture of manure.

Medicinal benefits

Cough and cold relief

Tulsi's anti-microbial and anti-inflammatory properties help relieve cough and cold symptoms.

In case of Bronchitis and Asthma, it helps soothe respiratory ailments like bronchitis and asthma. Boiled Tulsi leaf extract can soothe a sore throat.

Helps fight stress and mental health

Tulsi is considered an adaptogen, helping the body cope with stress and restore normal function. Tulsi improves cognitive function and memory.

Improves digestion

Tulsi can improve digestion and bowel movements. It is also known to help relieve gastrointestinal problems.

Regulates blood sugar and blood pressure

Tulsi can help lower blood sugar levels and improve insulin sensitivity. It can help lower LDL (bad cholesterol) levels. And also helps improve blood pressure.

Holy Basil is cultivated at many temples and the woody stems of plants that have died are used to make beads for sacred japa mala (rosaries). The beginning of the Hindu wedding season is marked by a festival known as Tulsi Vivah, in which homes and temples ceremonially wed holy basil to Vishnu. Water infused with the leaves is often given to the dying persons to help elevate their souls and funeral pyres are commonly offered Holy Basil twigs with the hope that the deceased may obtain moksha and be liberated from the cycle of rebirth.

27 Indian Asparagus

Scientific name: *Asparagus racemosus willd*
In English: Indian Asparagus
Konkani: Shatavari

Indian Asparagus, is believed to promote fertility and have a range of health benefits. It is also called a female friendly herb. The herb is thought to be adaptogenic, which means that it may help to regulate the body's systems and improve resistance to stress.

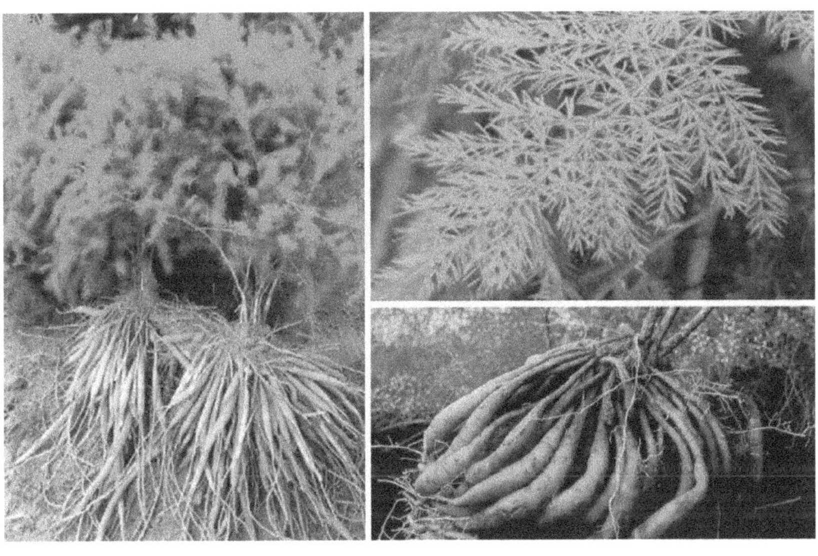

What is used - root

Propagation - Sow Indian Asparagus seeds in raised beds of 30 to 40 cm in width and 1-2 m length. After sowing, cover beds with thin cloth retain moisture. Seeds germinate within 10 days and seedlings are ready for transplanting when they attain the height of 40 cm.

Medicinal benefits

Increase breast milk production in mothers

Indian Asparagus is very useful in lactating mothers, especially those who have the problem of inadequate production of breast milk. It is traditionally used in Ayurvedic medicines to increase the breast milk.

Half a teaspoon of Shatavari powder is consumed with milk after lunch or dinner.

Managing heavy menstrual bleeding

Indian Asparagus is a common herb useful in managing gynaecological disorders in women, like unusual uterine or heavy menstrual bleeding. It also helps to restore the hormonal imbalance

Managing Stomach Ulcers

Indian Asparagus helps to manage stomach ulcers as hyperacidity is one of the primary causes of stomach ulcers. Its powder helps to reduce the acid level in the stomach and helps in quick healing.

Reduce Anxiety

Indian Asparagus is useful to manage the anxiety and has a calming effect on the body.

28. Indian Gooseberry

Scientific name: *Phyllanthus emblica*
In English: Indian gooseberry
Konkani: Avalo

Indian Gooseberry yields small berries round and yellow-green in colour. Though they are quite sour in taste their flavour can enhance some vegetable recipes and curries. Avalo has numerous medical benefits, which include boosting immunity, supporting heart and liver health, improving digestion and promoting healthy skin and hair. It has high Vitamin C content and anti-oxidant properties. Avalo is used in Goan homes to prepare chutneys, pickles and added to various vegetable dishes. Some people also add it to daals and rice and in south India it is used to prepare rasam.

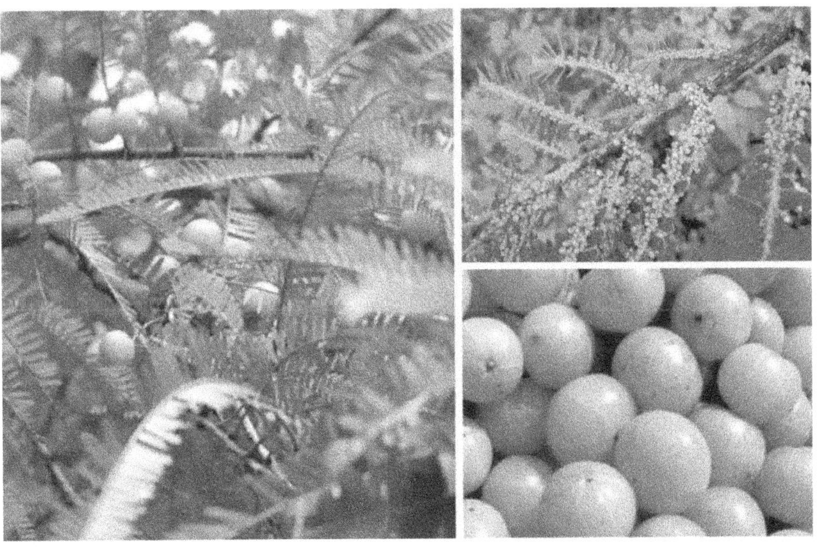

What is used - fruit

Propagation - Avalo is typically propagated by grafting and cuttings. Seed propagation is possible, but it results in low quality fruit and takes a longer time.

Medicinal benefits

Controlling blood sugar/Diabetes

Indian Gooseberry fruit contains soluble fibre and dissolves quickly in the body, which helps to slow the rate of absorbing sugar in the body. This can help reduce blood sugar spikes. Indian Gooseberry also has a beneficial effect on blood glucose and lipid counts in people with type 2 diabetes.

Boosting Immunity

Indian Gooseberry is one of the richest sources of Vitamin C. This high Vitamin C content enhances immunity, cell function and therefore helping the body fight infections & illnesses. Indian Gooseberry is also known to have anti-bacterial and anti-inflammatory properties.

Improving Digestion

The fibre in Indian Gooseberry helps to regulate bowel movements and may help to relieve from the condition like irritable bowel. High levels of Vitamin C in Indian Gooseberry berries helps body absorb nutrients from the food.

Weight Management

Since Indian Gooseberry is rich in fibre, it helps to feel full, when consumed with regular food, which may help reduce overall calorie intake.

Enhance Memory

Indian Gooseberry is known to enhance brain functioning, the anti-oxidants in Indian Gooseberry help in improving memory and cognitive function.

Hair Care

Indian Gooseberry is often used in hair oils to strengthen hair, reduce hair loss and improve scalp health.

Indian Gooseberry has been mentioned in most Ayurvedic practices for over a thousand years. It's a key ingredient in Chyawanprash, a popular Ayurvedic tonic to build immunity against colds, coughs and other infections.

One of the easiest ways to use Indian Gooseberry into diet is by juicing it. It can mix with fruits or vegetables to prepare nutritious drinks.

29 Indian devil tree or dita tree

Scientific name: *Alstonia scholaris (L.) R. Br*
In English: Indian devil tree or dita tree
Konkani: Saton

The Indian Devil Tree is renowned for its fragrant, greenish-white flowers and use in traditional medicine. It has been traditionally used in various medicines for treating a range of ailments, including fever, dysentery, diarrhoea, and respiratory issues. The bark and leaves contain compounds with potential anti-malarial, anti-inflammatory and anti-microbial properties. The Indian Devil Tree is a tall evergreen tree, sometimes grows to a height of 40 meters. It has a dark grey bark and glossy, dark green leaves. The tree's name "devil's tree" comes from the belief that it possesses magical powers or its strong fragrance is associated with supernatural force

What is used - bark, leaves

Propagation - It can be propagated by seeds or cuttings. Seeds should be sown in a well-drained soil and kept moist. Stem cuttings from healthy, mature plants can be rooted in a soil.

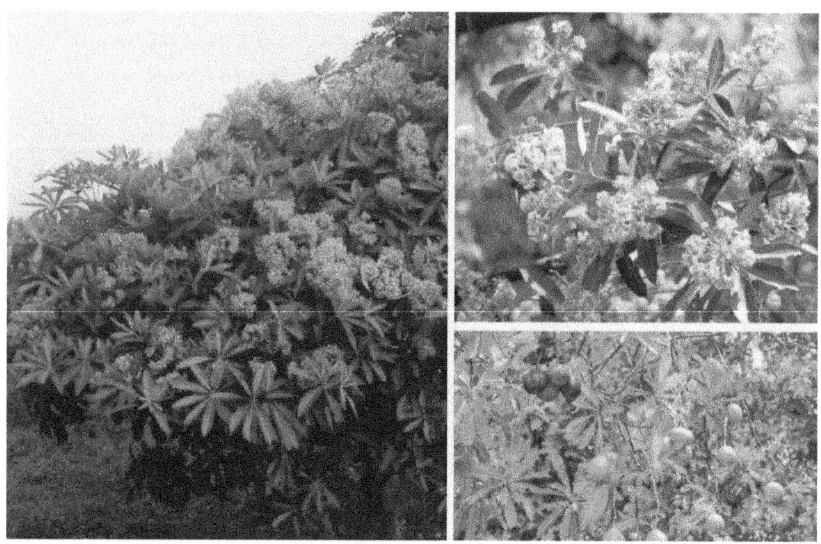

Medicinal benefits

Respiratory issues

It's used in the treatment of dyspnoea (difficulty breathing) and may also be helpful for bronchitis and asthma.

Reduce fever

The tree is used to reduce fever and is considered particularly effective in treating malarial fever.

Gastro-intestinal problems

Traditional uses include treating diarrhoea, dysentery and other gastro-intestinal issues.

Skin diseases

The juice of the leaves and bark preparations is used for various skin conditions, including ulcers, sores and inflammation.

The tree has been used in traditional systems for treating a variety of ailments, including beriberi, dropsy and liver congestion. The latex is used as a purgative.

30 Indian Hog Plum

Scientific name: *Spondias pinnata*
In English: Indian Hog Plum.
Konkani: Ambado

The Indian hog plum, is a tropical fruit native to Goa and other parts of India. It is a small, green and tart fruit with a tang taste used in Goan cuisine for chutneys, pickles and curry. The tree is a deciduous plant shedding its leaves seasonally. The fruit is oval or round with a green skin that turns yellowish-brown when ripe. It has a thin, shiny peel and a leathery skin.

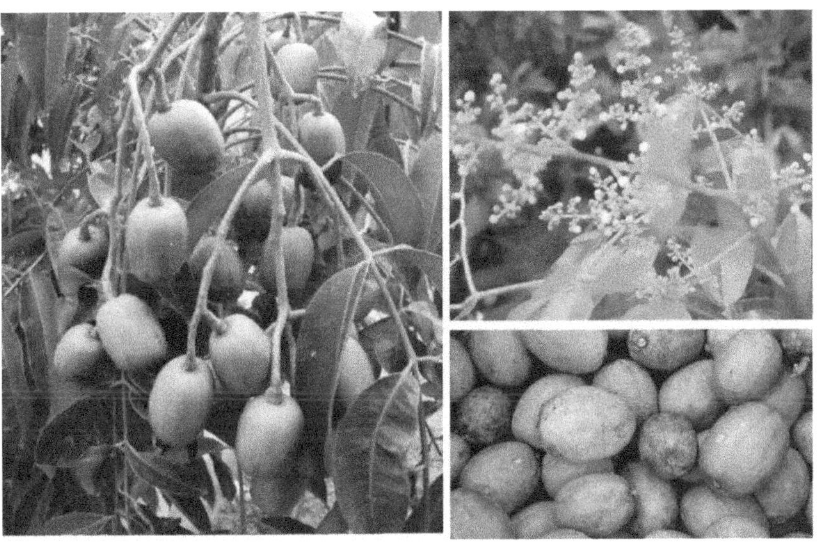

What is used - Fruit, Bark of tree

Propagation - It can be propagated by seeds or cuttings. Seeds should be sown in a well-drained soil and kept moist

Medicinal benefits

Digestive health

Indian Hog Plum fruit has high fibre content, which aids in digestion and maintaining a healthy gut.

Boosts immunity

Hog Plum is rich in anti-oxidants, which can help combat oxidative stress and potentially reduce the risk of chronic diseases. Hog Plum is a good source of vitamins A & C and iron.

Heart Health

Potassium and fibre in the fruit help regulate blood pressure and lower cholesterol levels, potentially reducing the risk of cardiovascular disease and stroke.

Anti-Inflammatory and Anti-Parasitic Effects

The bark extract helps protect against inflammation and the seeds may help suppress certain parasites.

In Goa, Indian Hog Plum is used to make pickles, is also added to curries and other vegetable dishes because of its sour taste. Once ripe and yellow it can be consumed directly and it has a tangy taste.

31 Indian Sarsaparilla

Scientific name: *Hemidesmus indicus (L.) R.Br*
In English: Indian Sarsaparilla
Konkani: Dudhshiri

The Indian Sarsaparilla root is known all over the world for its healing properties. It helps the body make more urine and sweat more. It can also help relieve fluid retention, puffiness or swelling and stomach bloating. It is traditionally used for its anti-inflammatory, anti-oxidant and detoxifying properties.

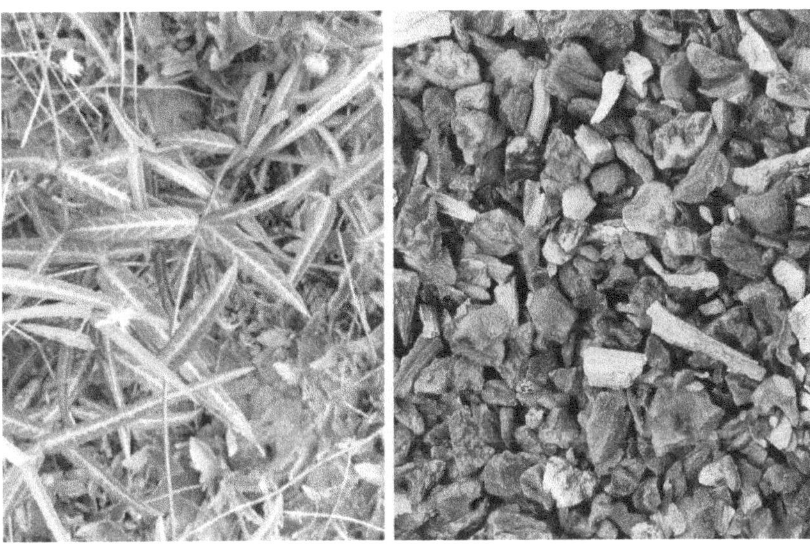

What is used - root

Propagation

The propagation and conservation of this Indian sarsaparilla traditionally take place by seeds. It can also be propagated by stem and root stock cuttings.

Medicinal benefits

Skin health

Indian Sarsaparilla is believed to have anti-oxidant, anti-inflammatory, and anti-microbial properties that can help treat various skin conditions like acne, pimples, psoriasis and eczema. It also promotes skin health and helps with conditions like dermatitis and leprosy.

Digestive health

It helps improve digestion and metabolism, potentially aiding in weight management.

It also reduces gas build-up and prevents bloating and constipation. It is also known to relieve digestive problems like diarrhoea and dysentery.

Kidney and Liver health

It's traditionally used for its detoxifying properties, which supports kidney and liver function. It helps remove toxins from the body and potentially improves overall health.

Boosting immune system

It's traditionally used as a blood purifier, potentially aiding in removing toxins from the blood.

32 Indian snakeroot

Scientific name: *Rauvolfia serpentine (L.) Benth. ex Kurz*
In English: Indian snakeroot
Konkani: Aatki

Indian snakeroot, also known as *Sarpagandha* in Hindi, is an evergreen shrub found in marshy areas. It has several Medicinal benefits, primarily due to its high concentration of reserpine, an alkaloid that helps control blood pressure. But this needs to be taken with caution as there could be serious side effects.

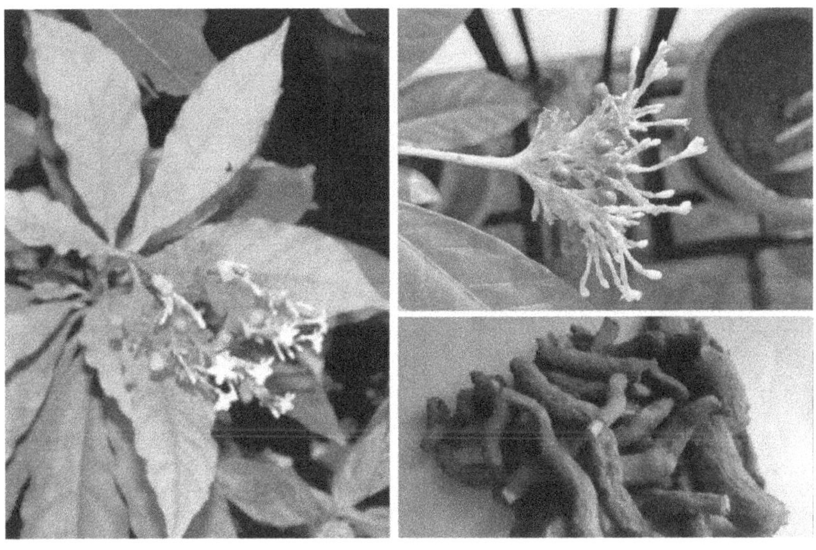

What is used – root

Propagation – can be propagated via seed, stem cutting or root cutting. For commercial plantation, seed propagation is the best.

Medicinal benefits

Controlling high blood pressure

Indian Snakeroot contains reserpine, which helps lower blood pressure and is a component in some hypertension medications.

Reduce stress and anxiety

The plant's sedative and blood pressure lowering properties contribute to its use in reducing stress and anxiety.

Relief from Insomnia

Chewing the root or consuming it can help soothe the mind and alleviate insomnia.

Stomach Issues

The plant can help cleanse the stomach and improve its function, potentially treating conditions like constipation and diarrhoea.

Treating skin issues

The plant is also used for treating skin conditions like acne, boils and eczema due to its anti-bacterial and anti-fungal properties.

In addition to the above traditional uses, Indian snakeroot is also used in some modern pharmaceutical formulations, for the treatment of hypertension and psychosis.

33 Java Plum

Scientific name: *Syzygium cumini*
In English: Java Plum
Konkani: Jambal

Java Plum, also known as Jamun or Indian blackberry, is an evergreen tree, which can grow 8 to 12 m tall. Its flowers are numerous, small, scented and dull white in color. The fruit is globose berry, which is dark purplish and becomes darker when it ripens. It has a seed in the middle which is roundish and smooth. It offers several Medicinal benefits due to its rich nutritional content and bioactive compounds

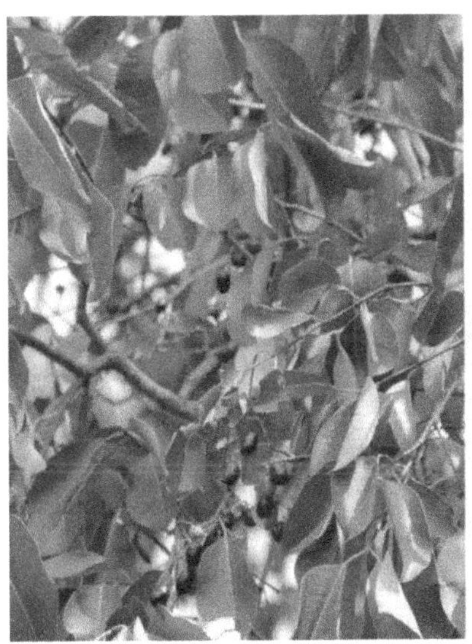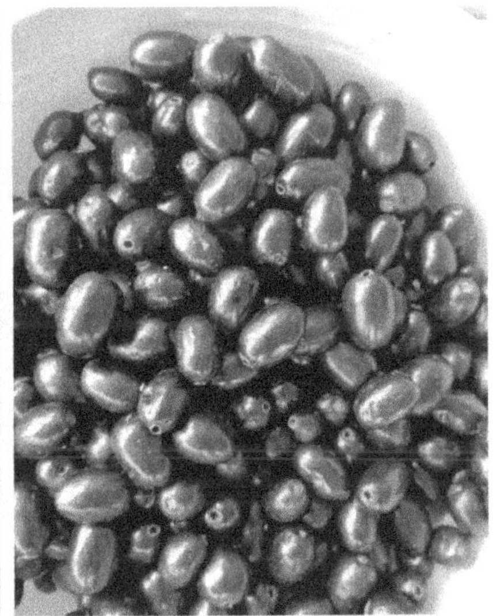

What is used - Fruit, seed

Propagation

Using seed, plant the seeds in a well-draining, sterile mix, covering them lightly, and spraying water on seeds. Java Plum can also be propagated using cuttings - make the cut just below a node, remove lower leaves and plant in fertile soil.

Medicinal benefits

Blood Sugar regulation

Java Plum is known to help regulate blood sugar levels, making it beneficial for patients with diabetes. This is because of compounds like jamboline, which improve insulin sensitivity.

Digestion

The high fibre content in Java Plum helps in digestion and can help relieve constipation and other digestive issues. It also acts as a natural astringent, which can help manage diarrhoea.

Boosting Immunity

Java Plum is rich in Vitamin C and anti-oxidants, which are crucial for boosting the immune system. These nutrients can help protect the body from infections and reduce the risk of chronic illnesses.

Skin Health

The Vitamin C in Java Plum is essential for collagen synthesis, which contributes to skin elasticity and can help with skin spots. Java Plum oil, extracted from seeds, is used in skincare products for its moisturizing and rejuvenating properties.

Heart Health

Java Plum contains anti-oxidants, particularly polyphenols, which may help reduce the risk of cardiovascular diseases. It also contributes to managing cholesterol levels.

34 Kokum

Scientific name: *Garcinia indica*
In English: Kokum
Konkani: Bhiran

Kokum, is a tropical fruit-bearing tree native to the Western Ghats of India. It has a wide range of culinary, medicinal, and industrial applications. The fruit is small, bright crimson red and has a sour taste. It is used in various Indian curries and pickles as a souring agent. The dried rind is used as a spice and is known for its flavor and cooling properties. In Goa, in summer, people love the cooling summer drink called kokum sharbat.

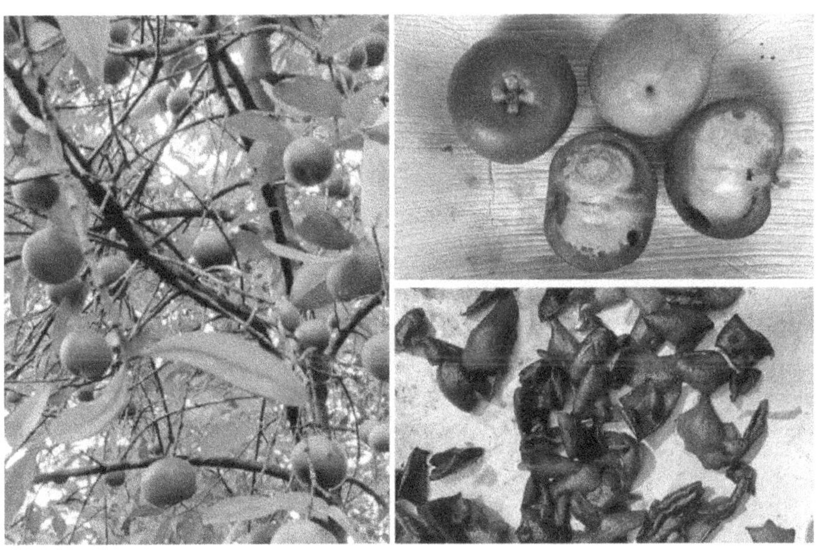

What is used - fruit

Propagation

Kokum is typically propagated through seeds and less commonly by grafting. Seed propagation involves collecting ripe fruits, extracting seeds and sowing directly in soil or poly bags for transplanting.

Medicinal benefits

Natural Cooling Agent

Kokum juice or syrup can provide a refreshing cooling effect, especially during hot summers.

Boosting Immunity

Kokum is rich in Vitamin C content, which helps boost the immune system. Kokum is rich in anti-oxidants, which help neutralize free radicals in the body. These anti-oxidants help reduce inflammation and lower the risk of chronic diseases like heart disease and cancer.

Promotes Digestive Health

Kokum can help relieve acidity, indigestion and other digestive issues. It contains hydroxycitric acid which promotes the secretion of digestive enzymes, thus helping in digestion. Kokum isalso known to reduce inflammation in stomach lining and prevent ulcers.

Diabetes Management

Kokum's anti-oxidant and anti-diabetic properties may help control blood sugar levels.

Weight Management

The compounds in kokum can suppress appetite and promote fat oxidation, potentially aiding in weight loss. It may also help reduce cholesterol and triglyceride levels, which can contribute to weight gain.

35 Lime

Scientific name: *Citrus aurantiifolia*
In English: Lime
Konkani: Limbu

The Lime fruit is a key ingredient in certain pickles and chutneys, and lime juice is used to flavour drinks and foods. Lime soda is a favourite drink of every Goan. The juice of lime fruits may be concentrated, dried, frozen, or canned. Citrate of lime and citric acid are also prepared from fruits. The tree seldom grows to 5 m height and if not pruned becomes shrub. Its branches spread, with small leaves and many small sharp thorns. The evergreen leaves are pale green and it bears small white flowers, which are usually borne in clusters.

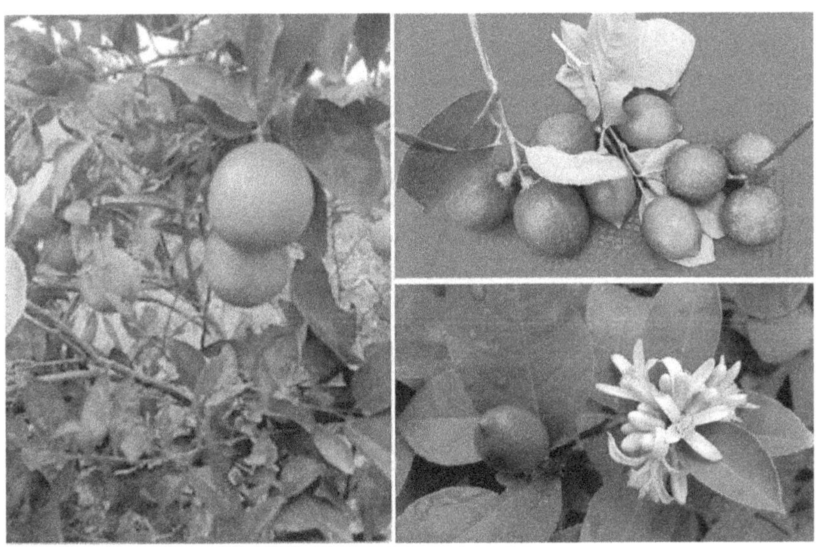

What is used - fruit

Propagation - Lemon trees are commonly propagated by cuttings, a simple and effective method where a healthy branch is cut, treated with rooting hormone and planted in soil to develop roots. However, the grafting method has become more popular in the recent years.

Medicinal benefits

Prevents Infection

Lime has high levels of Vitamin C that helps protect from infection and speed up body's healing process.

Reduce Inflammation

Lime contains anti-oxidants, which helps reduce inflammation and even help prevent certain chronic illnesses. This means some relief in case of Arthritis and other joint problems.

Prevent Kidney Stones

Lime helps keep Kidney Stones at bay. The citric acid in lemons and other citrus fruits makes it more difficult for kidney stones to form.

Improve Immune Health

As Lime contains Vitamin C, which is vital for immune health, regularly consuming limes can even help prevent the common cold.

Improves Digestion

Drinking lime water improves digestion. Limes are acidic in nature and help saliva break down food for better digestion. Additionally, the compounds in Lime stimulate secretion of digestive juices. In case of constipation, the acidity of Limes can clear the excretory system and stimulate bowel activity. And for frequent heartburn or acid reflux, drinking a glass of warm water with 2 teaspoons of lime juice about 30 minutes before meals helps prevent reflux symptoms.

Helps in Weight Loss

Another benefit of lime water/soda is to reduce weight. Citric acids can boost metabolism, helping in burning more calories and store less fat.

Limes have many uses. Everyone loves a refreshing lime soda. It is also used as seasoning salads and various meats. Lime is also found in soaps, which is more effective to wash off dirt and wax.

36. Malabar nut

Scientific name: *Justicia adhatoda*
In English: Malabar nut
Konkani: Adulsa

The Adhathoda means 'untouched by goats' in Tamil because of the bitter taste of the leaves. Adulsa grows as a shrub with leaves that are 9 to10 cm in length and about 4 to 5 cm wide. It often grown as an edge plant, on the boundaries and its leaves and twigs are utilized as green-manure. The whole plant or its roots, leaves, bark and flowers are used in various herbal preparations. Its flowers are usually white and show large, dense, axillary spikes. Its fruits when young appear like club-shaped capsules.

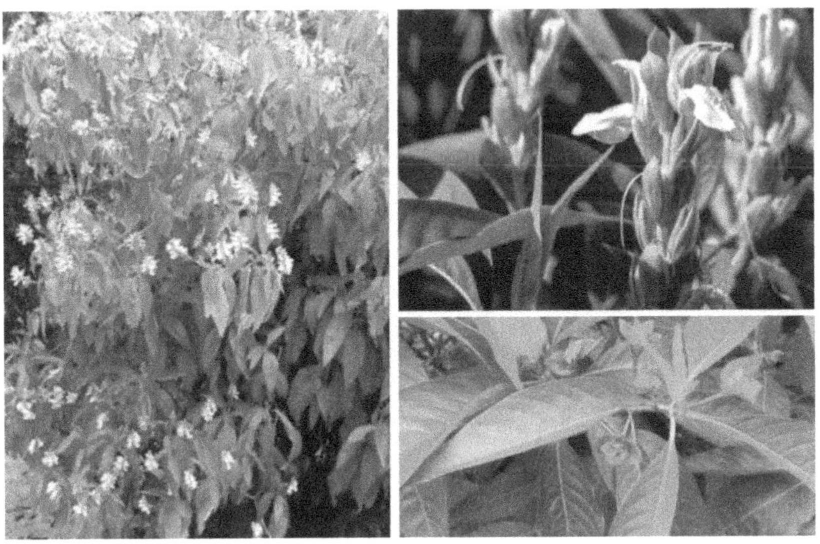

What is used - leaves, branches and stems.

Propagation - Adulsa is primarily propagated by stem cuttings. Seed propagation is possible, but is less reliable due to low germination rates. About 15 to 20 cm long stem cuttings are made, with at least 3-4 nodes, and the cuttings are then planted in pots or directly in the soil.

Medicinal benefits

Cough and Cold Relief - Adulsa is widely regarded as an excellent remedy to soothe coughs and colds, and its leaves are known to relieve respiratory congestion. In most Goan homes there is Adulsa cough syrup, which is an extract from the leaves. Steam inhalation is prepared of Adulsa leaves, which helps in loosening the mucus in the lungs and clearing the respiratory tract.

In case of sore throat, leaves are boiled to make a tea that helps to ease the irritation and inflammation of the throat. In Goan households, if one member of the family gets a cold then other members also have the adulsa tea, with a little honey to neutralize the bitter taste, as a preventive measure.

Reducing Fever - In addition to relieving cough and cold, Adulsa leaves are also boiled in water and are used to take bath to reduce high fever.

Blood purification - Adulsa helps to clear the clots and blockages in the arteries, which in turn prevents heart attacks. The medicinal plant also regulates blood pressure levels, which further aids with heart health.

Relief from wounds/cuts and also Skin infections

For a cut/wound to heal quickly collagen needs to be created. Adulsa promotes the production of collagen, basically crush some Adulsa leaves, and apply them directly to the wound to see the magical healing powers.

Reduce inflammation

Adulsa's leaves have strong anti-inflammatory properties that can help reduce joint pain and inflammation from conditions like arthritis, especially in older people.

Helps with Digestive Health

Adulsa's leaves are also known to promote digestion and has anti-ulcer properties. The plant is also rich in anti-oxidants, which supports overall health and wellness.

The Adulsa leaves are a power-house of natural healing with multiple benefits. In today's world Adulsa is available either as a capsule or a syrup making it easy to take advantage of the health benefits of the Adulsa plant.

37 Mango

Scientific name: *Mangifera indica*
In English: Mango
Konkani: Ambo

What is used - fruit, leaves

Propagation - There are three methods of propagation - by seed, air layering and grafting.

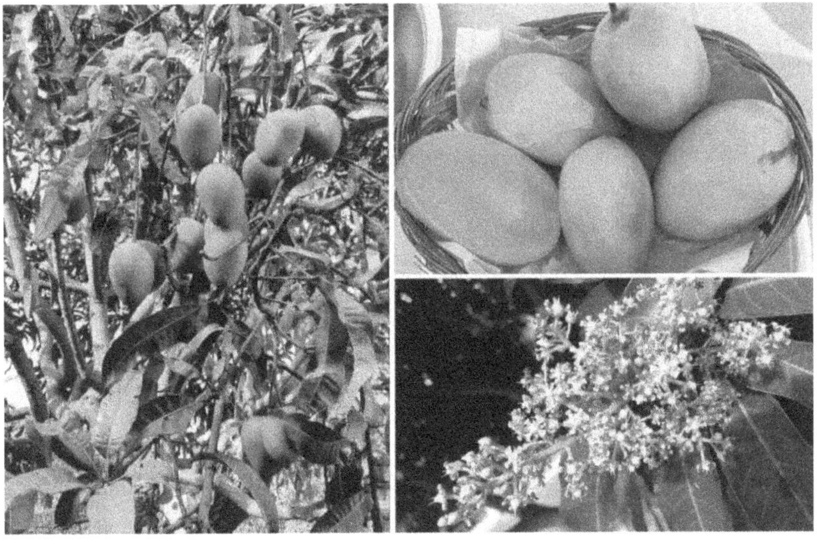

Medicinal benefits

Support gut health

Mangoes are good source of both soluble and insoluble fibre. Fibre is a carbohydrate in plant food that cannot be digested. Insoluble fibre doesn't break down in digestive tract, which adds bulk to a stool and is easier to pass.

Regular intake of mango leaf infusion acts as a stomach tonic, flushing out toxins from the body and helping prevent various stomach ailments such as stomach ulcers and digestive disorders. Prepare mango leaf tea by boiling 10-15 fresh mango leaves.

Control blood pressure

Most people aren't getting enough potassium, a mineral that helps counteract the effects of sodium in body. Excess sodium and less potassium can cause high blood pressure (hypertension). Potassium helps fight high blood pressure, which is a major risk factor for heart disease and stroke. Eating mangoes and other potassium-rich foods each day can boost cardiovascular health.

Helps with Weight loss

Mangoes may help control hunger, which could help to stick to healthy eating habits. Mangoes take longer to digest than low-fibre foods and feel fuller for longer, without consuming much of calories.

Prevent tooth decay

Mango leaves can be used for cleaning teeth for dental and oral health as it has anti-bacterial activity.

38 Moringa

Scientific name: *Moringa oleifera*
In English: Moringa
Konkani: Mashinga

Moringa, also known as the miracle tree, boasts numerous Medicinal benefits. In addition, Moringa has numerous applications in cooking. In Goa a simple vegetable is prepared using the leaves, onion and coconut. It is also commonly added to broth to make a simple soup.

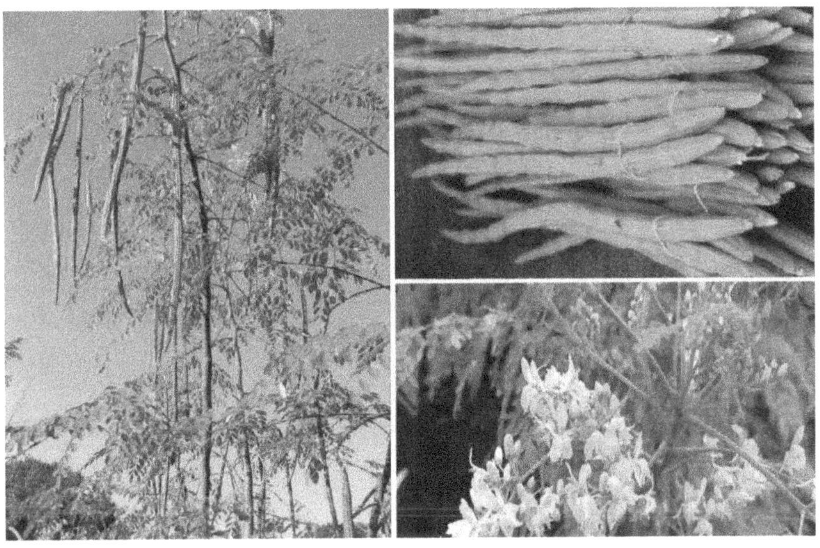

What is used - Leaves

Propagation - Moringa is easily propagated by stem cuttings and seeds.

Medicinal benefits

Helps in body immunity and clean skin

Moringa contains powerful anti-oxidants that can help protect the body against damage caused by free radicals, which helps boost body immunity and glow of skin.

Moringa has anti-inflammatory properties that can help reduce inflammation in the body. It also has anti-microbial properties that can help fight off infections caused by bacteria, fungi and viruses. Moringa leaves can be steeped in hot water to make a refreshing tea.

Healing cuts and wounds

Moringa can promote faster wound healing and reduce the risk of infection

Regulate blood sugar

Moringa helps lower blood sugar levels and improve insulin sensitivity, helping in regulating blood sugar levels in diabetic patients.

Heart Health

Moringa also helps lower blood pressure, which is beneficial for cardiovascular health. Moringa has also been linked to other potential benefits, including improved liver function, reduced cholesterol levels, and improved digestion.

Moringa can be consumed in powder form and is also available capsules.

39 Neem

Scientific name: *Azadirachta indica*
In English: Neem
Konkani: Kodu-limbu

Neem is a fast-growing tree, and is valued as a medicinal plant, a source of organic pesticides, and also for its timber. Neem trees in Goa can reach 15 to 20 m in height .The leaves are serrated and are evergreen. The fruit is yellow-green and has a sweet-flavoured pulp. The plant is hardy and resilient and grows well in poor, rocky soils, as well as the tropical climate of Goa. It is also called the village pharmacy.

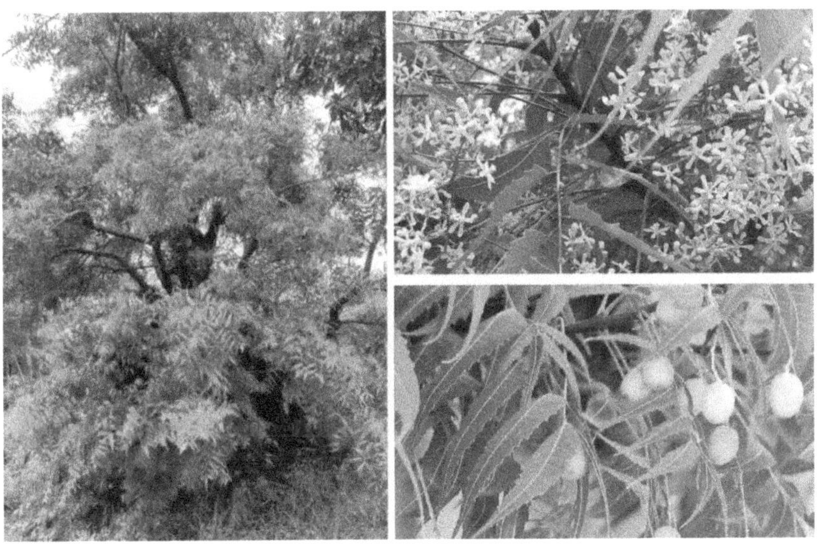

What is used - leaves, branches

Propagation - The tree is easily propagated by seeds.

Medicinal benefits

Used for dental and oral health

Chewing neem bark/branches to promote oral hygiene was a common practice in the past generations. Neem has antiseptic, anti-inflammatory, antioxidant compounds, which are good for boosting immunity and promoting oral health.

Diabetes management

Neem leaves are bitter in taste. Boiling neem leaves in water for 10 minutes and consuming it helps regulate the blood sugar level as it revives cells that produce insulin to maintain blood sugar levels

Helps with liver and kidney health

Neem has anti-oxidant and anti-inflammatory properties, which help fight oxidative stress, which in turn promote liver and kidney health. Oxidative stress is caused by building unstable molecules called free radicals. Although body naturally produces free radicals as a by-product of metabolism, external sources increase their presence and neem tea can help regulate these free radicals.

Treat Acne

Neem is used to treat acne, reduce blemishes, and improve skin elasticity. There are many Acne face washes and rubs prepared from neem extract.

Nearly all parts of the Neem tree are useful. Many of its medicinal and cosmetic uses are based on anti-bacterial and anti-fungal properties. Neem is commonly used in shampoos for treating dandruff, in soaps, creams for skin conditions and acne. It can also be found in some toothpastes and mouthwashes.

40 Nutmeg

Scientific name: *Myristica fragrans*
In English: Nutmeg
Konkani: Zaiphol

The word Nutmeg comes from the Latin words nux - meaning nut, and meg - meaning musky. Nutmeg has been used for centuries to add flavor and aroma to many dishes. The seed is dark brown, ovoid and about 2 to 3 cm long.

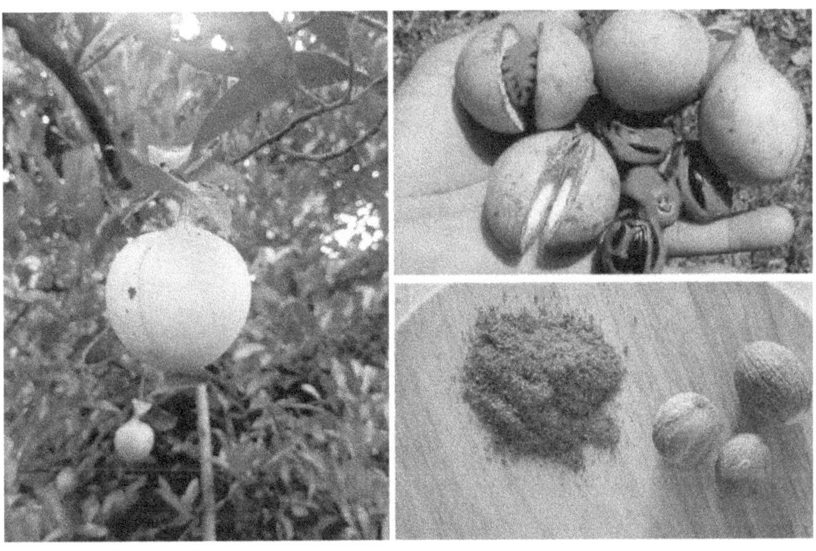

What is used - seed

Propagation

Nutmeg can be propagated by both seeds and vegetative methods, with grafting being the most common commercial practice. Grafting is preferred for maintaining the desirable traits of high-yielding varieties.

Medicinal benefits

Digestive Support

Nutmeg has properties that can help relieve bloating, gas, and constipation. It helps stimulate digestive enzymes, improving metabolism and potentially aiding in weight loss.

Boosts Immunity

Nutmeg contains anti-inflammatory compounds that may help reduce inflammation throughout the body. The anti-oxidant properties can protect against cell damage caused by free radicals, supporting overall health. Nutmeg is also known to improve sleep quality.

Oral Health

Nutmeg has anti-bacterial compounds, which may help prevent dental cavities and gum problems.

Improves Brain Function

Nutmeg contains essential oils with neuroprotective properties that may enhance cognitive function, improve memory and protect against age-related cognitive decline.

Potential for Weight Management

Nutmeg helps boost metabolism and curb appetite and reduce weight loss. It can also be used to relieve stress and anxiety.

Nutmeg is used in baked goods, confectionaries, puddings, meats, sauces, vegetables and beverages. It contains psychoactive chemicals that can cause hallucinations, confusion, drowsiness, incoherent speech and therefore it is important to use it in moderation.

41 Onion

Scientific name: *Allium cepa*
In English: Onion
Konkani: Kaṇdo

Onion is primarily cultivated as a vegetable and is widely used in Goan homes for curry, vegetables and also meats. It is mostly fried with garlic, and other spices to give the dish a taste. The bulb is commonly consumed, but the spathe and leaves are also edible.

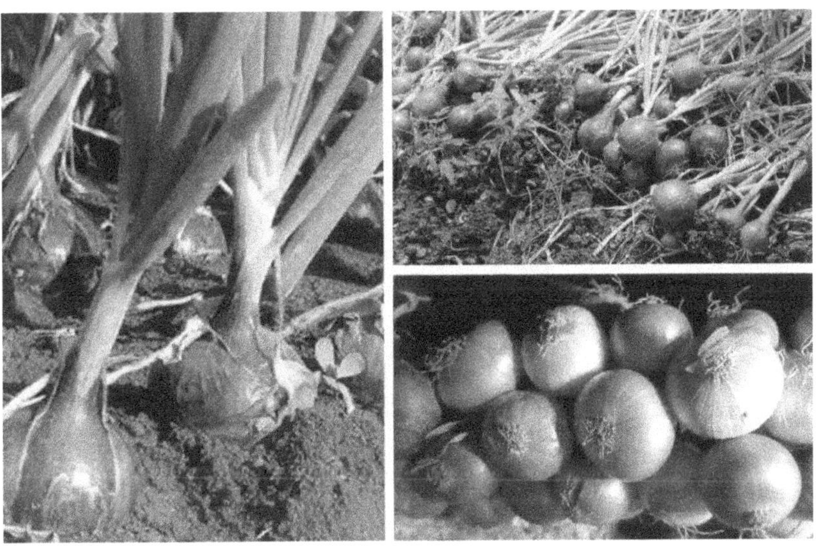

What is used - root/bulb

Propagation - The most common method of propagation is by seeds and bulbs where seedlings are raised in a nursery bed and then transplanted to the main field.

Medicinal benefits

Improve Digestive Health

Onions have compounds that act as prebiotics, which is food for gut's healthy bacteria, which helps in digestion. Diseases ranging from diabetes, colon cancer and depression have been linked to not having enough healthy gut bacteria.

Boosting immunity

Anti-oxidant compounds help prevent cell damage in the body. Anti-oxidants, found in onions, protect health in several ways, which include fighting inflammation and boosting the immune system. Onions are also a good source of vitamins, minerals, and fibre. Drinking onion water concentrate can also help fight cold and flu symptoms.

Reduce risk of heart disease

Onions contain organic sulphur compounds, which give them their strong taste and smell. These compounds help reduce the level of cholesterol in body and help break down blood clots, lowering risk of heart disease and stroke. Eating onions raw in a salad, rather than cooking, is good for the availability of sulphur compounds.

Regulate blood sugar

The compounds in Onion are known to boost insulin production, making them a helpful vegetable choice for diabetes.

42 Indian Rennet tree

Scientific name: *Withania coagulans*
In English: Paneer seeds
Konkani: Paneer biyo

Paneer Seeds also called Indian Rennet is a plant with both culinary and medicinal benefits. It is primarily known for its ability to coagulate milk and produce paneer. And is well known for its use in ayurvedic practices.

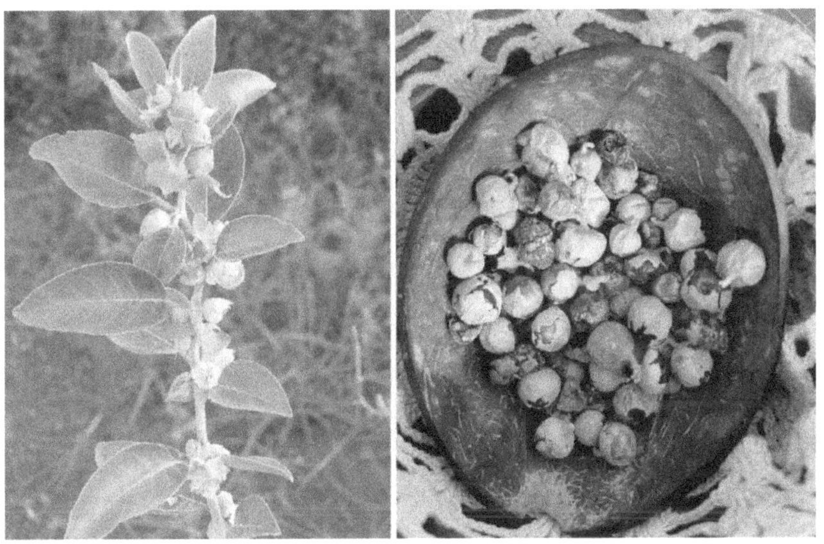

What is used - Seeds, fruit

Propagation - Paneer seeds are primarily propagated through seed germination but natural propagation is often challenging. Micro propagation or plant tissue culture, offers a more reliable and efficient method for mass production and conservation.

Medicinal benefits

Blood Sugar Management:

Paneer seeds help manage blood sugar levels and repair beta cells in the pancreas, which are responsible for insulin production. It improves insulin supply within the body, which is crucial for regulating blood sugar levels.

Wound healing

Possesses anti-platelet properties, which can help in improving wound healing process in diabetic patients.

Anti-oxidant properties

The paneer fruit can reduce oxidative stress and maintain anti-oxidant status, which can protect cells from damage.

Kidney protection

It may reduce pro-inflammatory symptoms in the kidneys, potentially mitigating the development and progression of renal injury in diabetes.

The seeds of the plant, along with its leaves and fruits, have been used for centuries to make a type of soft cheese called paneer in India.

43 Papaya

Scientific name: *Carica papaya*
In English: Papaya
Konkani: Popai

Papaya is a tropical fruit having commercial importance because of its high nutritive and medicinal value. The fruit being perishable, it should be consumed in a couple of days after ripening.

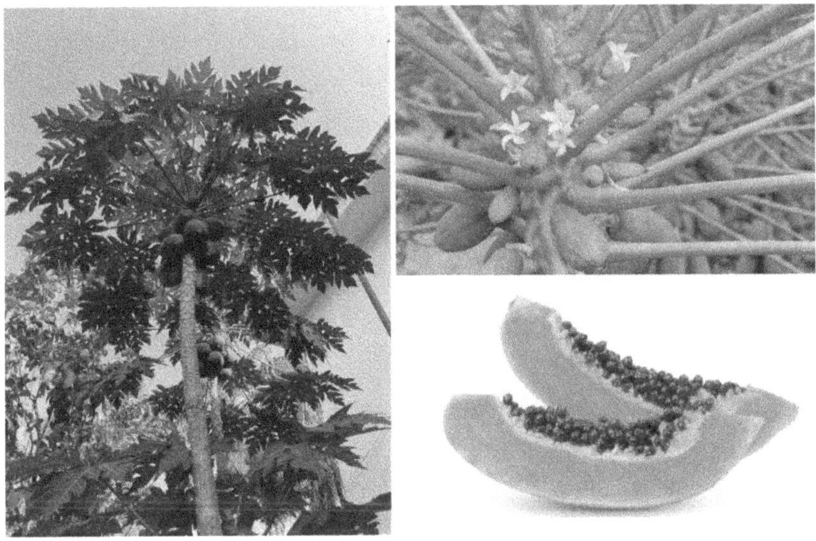

What is used - fruit

Propagation - Papaya is commercially propagated by seed and tissue culture plants, but the papaya found in the backyard of most Goan homes grow from seeds, thrown in wet soil.

Medicinal benefits

Helps in digestion

Papaya is high in fibre and water content, which help prevent constipation and promotes regulation and the health of the digestive tract.

Vision and eye health

Some of the organic compounds present in papaya help prevent inflammation and oxidative stress in age-related eye diseases, such as macular degeneration.

Preventing Asthma

Consuming a high number of fruits and vegetables lowers the risk of developing asthma and can prevent the worsening of asthama. This may be due to dietary components in fruits and vegetables, such as anti-oxidants, fibre, and Vitamin D. These nutrients can assist the immune system's typical functioning, which over-responds in people with asthma.

Improves Bone Health

Papaya is a source of vitamin K. Low intakes of Vitamin K is associated with higher risk of bone fracture. Thus, adequate Vitamin K consumption is important for good health. It improves calcium absorption and may reduce urinary excretion of calcium to strengthen and rebuild bones.

Regulating Sugar levels

People with type 1 diabetes who consume high fibre diets have lower blood glucose levels. In addition, high fibre diets have improved blood sugar, lipid and insulin levels.

Reducing risk of Heart disease

Anti-oxidants in papaya, such as lycopene, reduce the risk of heart disease and stroke. Papaya also contains fibre, which helps lower cholesterol. It is also high in potassium, which can be beneficial for those with high blood pressure. An increase in potassium intake along with a decrease in sodium intake is the most important dietary change someone can make to reduce their risk of cardiovascular disease.

44 Soursop

Scientific name: *Annona muricata*
In English: Soursop
Konkani: Patpanas

Soursop plant is a small evergreen plant native to Central and tropical South America and is grown in kitchen gardens of the backyard of most Goan households. Soursop fruits are large and oval-shaped, with green prickly exteriors and are 20 to 30 cm long. The fruit is mostly consumed raw and is known to have anti-cancer properties

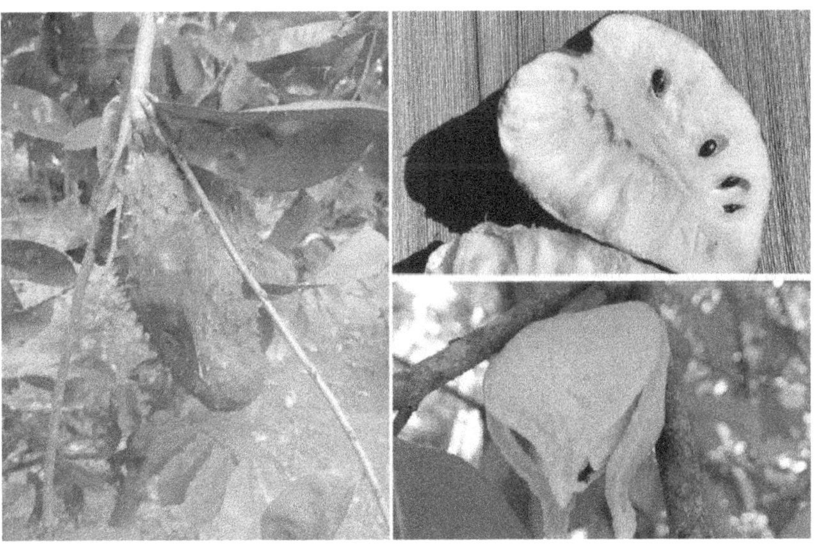

What is used - fruit, leaves

Propagation

Soursop is primarily propagated through seeds, but other methods like grafting and air layering are also popular. Soaking seeds in water for 24 hours helps in germination. Seeds should be sown in in pots or poly bags and   placed in a warm, shaded area. Germination can take about 15 to 30 days. Seedlings can be transplanted to field when they are about one foot in height.

Medicinal benefits

Anti-Cancer potential

Extracts from soursop leaves have potential anti-cancer effects, including the ability to kill cancer cells and reduce inflammation. It is effective against cancer cells.

Heart Health

Soursop contains potassium, which is crucial for regulating heart rhythm and blood pressure, potentially reducing the risk of cardio-vascular diseases.

Digestive Health

Soursop's fibre content can aid digestion, promote regular bowel movements and potentially reduce the risk of digestive disorders.

Boost body's Immune system

Soursop is rich in anti-oxidants and compounds with anti-inflammatory effects, which can help protect cells from damage and reduce inflammation in the body.

Soursop, particularly extracts and teas, have shown anti-bacterial and anti-parasitic properties, which help to fight infections.

In traditional medicine, Soursop has been used to treat various ailments, including cough, fever, headache, and insomnia. Also, a leaf extract is used to kill head lice and bedbugs.

45 Star Fruit

Scientific name: *Averrhoa carambola*
In English: Star fruit
Konkani: Carambola

Star fruit is a popular tropical fruit. The plant produces clusters of small, lilac-colored, bell-shaped flowers, which give way to oblong-shaped fruits with characteristic five-angled edges, resembling a starfish when sliced. The star fruit boasts a green to yellow hue with an attractive smooth waxy surface.

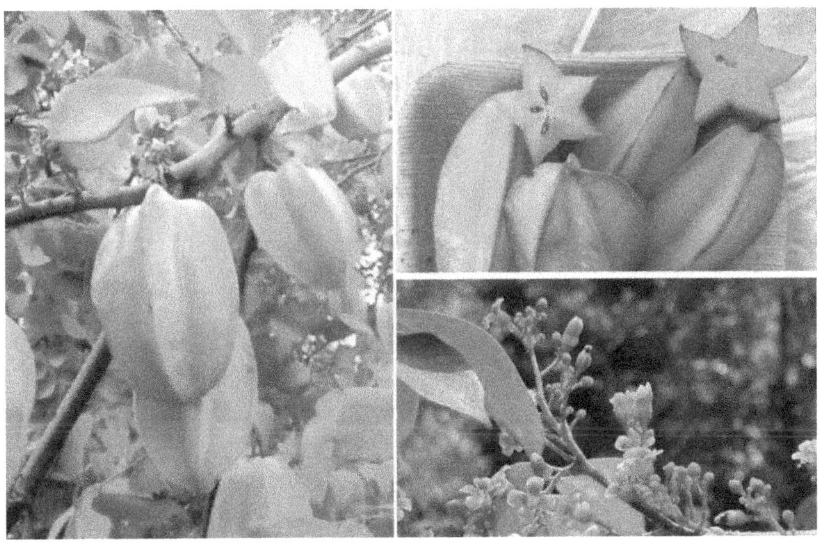

What is used - fruit

Propagation

Star fruit propagation can be achieved by seeds and grafting, where a branch from one tree is attached to the rootstock of another. Ripe, golden-yellow star fruit should be chosen for the best seed quality.

Medicinal benefits

Immune Support

Star fruit is rich in vitamin C and anti-oxidants, which is crucial for building and maintaining a healthy immune system. Vitamin C helps the body fight off infections and protects against free radical damage.

Improves Heart Health

Potassium in Star fruit can help lower blood pressure, which reduces the risk of heart attack or stroke. Fibre in star fruit may also help lower cholesterol levels.

Digestion and Bowel Health

Fibre in Star fruit promotes digestion by helping in regular bowel movements and preventing constipation.

Blood Sugar Regulation

Star fruit helps regulate blood sugar levels, which can be beneficial for individuals managing diabetes.

Weight Management

Star fruit is low in calories and high in fibre, making it a good option for weight management as it can help in feeling fuller for longer.

46 Sweet Flag

Scientific name: *Acorus calamus L.*
In English: Sweet Flag, Calamus
Konkani: Vaikhand

Sweet Flag is found in tropical and sub-tropical moist/water logged areas, close to water bodies and rivers, and is also cultivated in gardens and orchards in Goa. It is a perennial herb, growing with profusely branched rhizomes, having stout joints with large leaf scars. Leaves are simple, alternate, distichous, closely arranged. Flowers pale green, fragrant, arranged compactly on a sessile, cylindrical, short, stump. The fruits are pulpy and loaded with seeds.

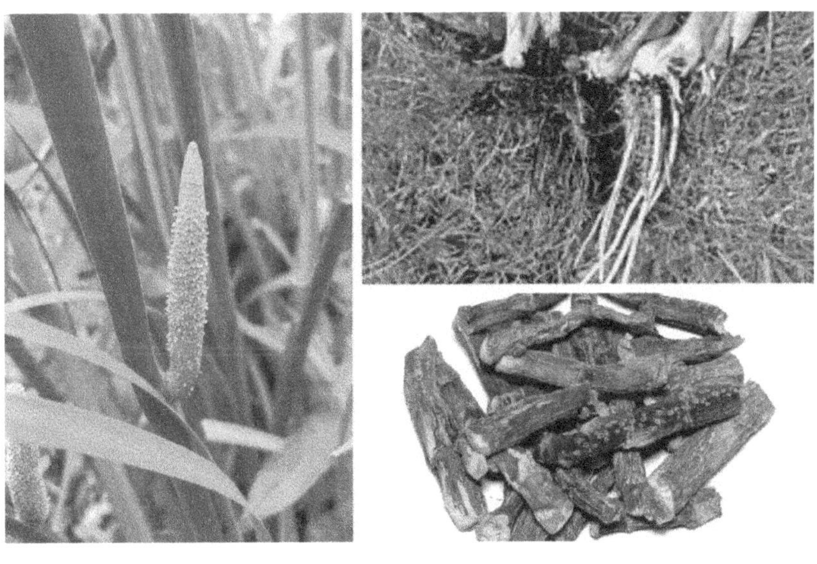

What is used - Rhizome (root)

Medicinal benefits

Helps with throat issues

Sweet flag is an excellent remedy for cold and it cures sore throat and cough.

Prevents pain, inflammation and infection

Sweet Flag (Vacha) oil application aids in preventing skin infections. It also relieves pain and swelling caused by arthritis or rheumatoid arthritis. These disorders have the potential to become very severe, impair mobility and alter lifestyle. This necessitates taking all preventive and curative measures that are available. When breathed, vacha also soothes the mind and relieves headaches.

Guards against head lice

Vacha oil is a natural insecticide and works well to get rid of lice. Applying it to the scalp has no negative effects because it is mild and safe for external usage. The most effective natural remedy to get rid of lice is the sweet flag.

Combats Epilepsy, Depression and Boosting Memory

Vacha is renowned for reducing anxiety and enhancing memory. It acts like a nerve tonic and aids in relaxation as well as for release of stress and despair. It has also been observed that pounded vacha root soaked in boiling hot water can benefit to cure epilepsy.

Helpful During Childbirth

Strong uterine contractions brought on by vacha aid in difficult or protracted labour. Enabling the mother to give birth to the kid with ease. Dysmenorrhea can be effectively treated with this herb as well.

Sweet Flag can also be used as a pesticide. They are safe to use around young children and help repel insects and cockroaches. Sweet Flag powder can be mixed in water and sprinkled in areas to repel insects.

47 Tamarind

Scientific name: *Tamarindus indica*
In English: Tamarind
Konkani: Chinch

Tamarind, with its sweet and sour taste, offers various health benefits, including acting as a natural laxative, boosting immunity with its anti-oxidant properties and potentially aiding in managing blood sugar and weight. The tree grows to about 24 m tall and has feather like leaves with leaflets that are about 2 cm long. The yellow flowers are borne in small clusters. The fruit is long and slender, about 7 to 24 cm long. It contains 1 to 12 large, flat seeds embedded in a soft brownish pulp.

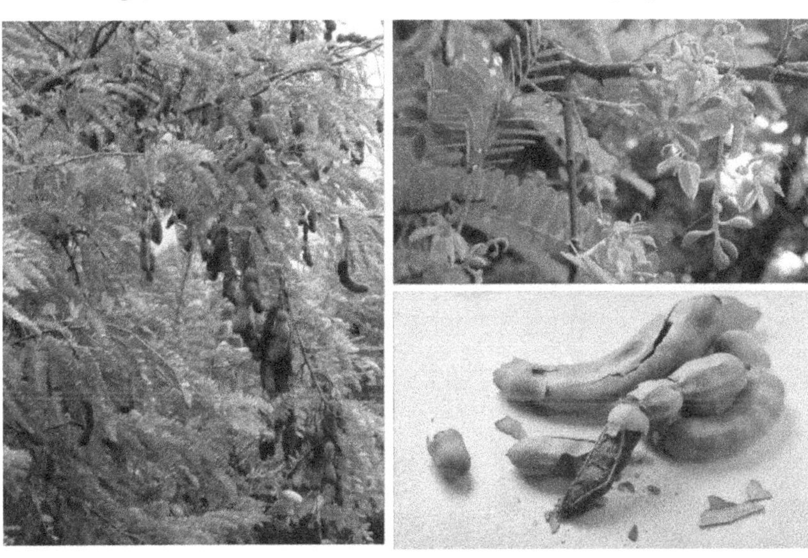

What is used - fruit

Propagation - Tamarind plants can be propagated by seeds and through vegetative methods like grafting. Seed propagation is the most common method, while grafting allows for faster growth and preservation of desired traits

Medicinal benefits

Improves body Immunity

Tamarind is rich in anti-oxidants and high in calcium, fibre and magnesium. Magnesium is an important nutrient that supports more than 300 essential processes in the body, including regulating nerve and muscle function, maintaining blood pressure and strong bones.

Anti-oxidants are naturally occurring chemicals found in some food. They help the body fight cellular damage from free radicals, unstable molecules that can cause oxidative stress and lead to disease and other health issues like autoimmune, cardio-vascular and inflammatory disease, cataracts, cancer, and neuro-degenerative disorders like alzheimers and parkinsons.

Reduce inflammation

Tamarind pulp is rich in potassium and other compounds that reduce inflammation. Reducing inflammation reduces the risk of short-term illness and chronic diseases.

Control diabetes

The patients with diabetes are familiar with the glycemic index and blood sugar.

Tamarind is relatively high in sugar, but is also low in glycemic index and doesn't cause spikes in blood sugar.

48 Tellicherry bark

Scientific name: *Holarrhena antidy-senterica (L.) Wall*
In English: Tellicherry bark
Konkani: Nagalkudo

The Tellicherry plant grows to a shrub or small tree with an average height of 4 to 8 m. The branched tree has a slightly pale bark, short stalk green leaves and white aromatic flowers that turn yellow with age. The fruits are cylindrical and generally crop up in pairs and seeds are light-brown. It can be used in treating dysentery, diarrhoea and intestinal worms and some studies also suggesting anti-inflammatory, anti-diabetic and anti-microbial properties

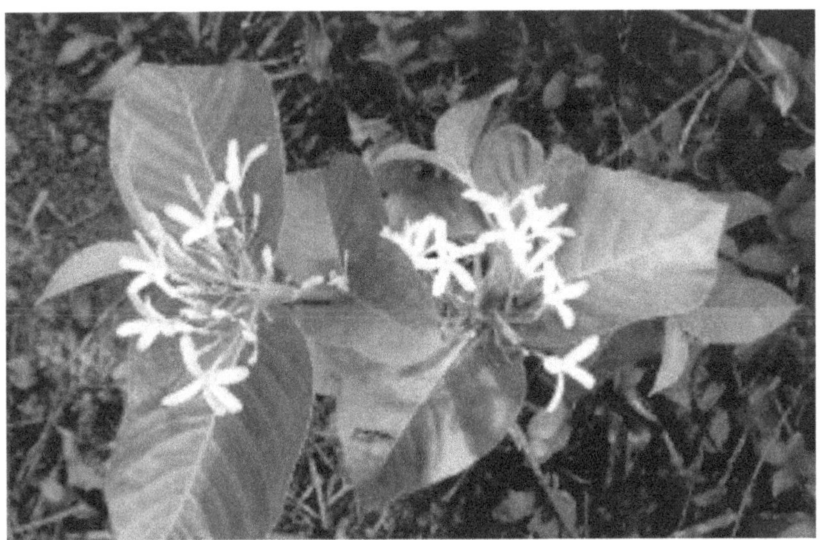

What is used - Stem, bark and seeds

Propagation - It is propagated through seeds or cuttings.

Medicinal benefits

Digestive Disorders

Both the bark and fruits of the plant are very useful in relieving digestive disorders like constipation, dysentery, diarrhoea, stomach aches and gas. In addition, it can be used to get rid of intestinal worms.

Reduce mouth ulcers

Extracts from the stem, bark and seeds of the herb contain certain salts and calcium that help relieve mouth ulcers.

Prevents loss of Appetite loss

In people regularly suffering from Appetite loss, this herb helps relieve appetite loss.

Tissue relief

The tonic properties help remove muscle weakness from the body and are also very useful in toning the vaginal tissues in women after delivery.

Healing Wounds

The bark and seeds of this plant are very useful in healing wounds.

49 Tinospora

Scientific name: *Tinospora cordifolia*
In English: Tinospora
Konkani: Gilloy

It is a climbing vine with several elongated twining branches with a papery bark. The vine is quick in spreading. The leaves are typically heart shaped and the flowers are yellow arising from the nodes. The fruits are drupes and turn red when ripe.

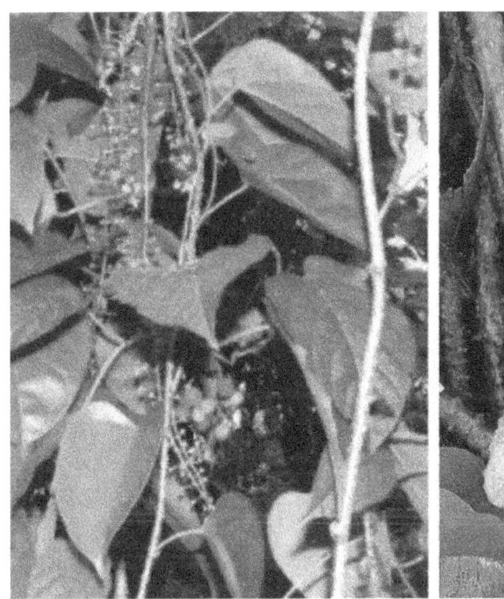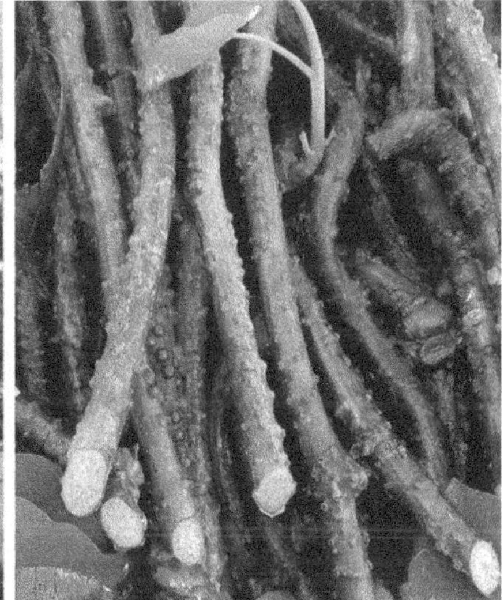

What is used - stem, leaves

Propagation - The stem cuttings with nodes are sown directly in the soil. The plant requires support to grow, which can be provided by raising wooden stakes or trellis or an already growing tree can be used for support.

Medicinal benefits

Reducing fevers

The fresh stem is used to prepare decoction for fevers. It also helps in reducing weakness caused by repeated fever.

Skin disorders

A fresh juice of Tinospora helps to treat different kinds of skin disorders.

Helps with Liver Disorders

A tonic of Tinospora or a vegetable curry made from leaves and stem can help to control jaundice.

Used as an aphrodisiac

The juice of Tinospora acts as an aphrodisiac.

Helps with Digestion

A simple vegetable curry made of the leaves and stem of Tinospora serves as a digestive tonic and promotes bowel movement and controls piles.

The stem and leaves are highly nutritive and can be used for hormonal imbalance, diabetes and soft tissue joints and bones (rheumatism).

50 Toothache tree

Scientific name: *Zanthoxylum rhetsum*
In English: Toothache tree
Konkani: Teflam/Telfala

The toothache tree in Goa is commonly known as Teflam. The dried husk of the fruit is a spice in Goan cuisine, known for its peculiar, pungent and tangy taste. The bark is grey and has cone-shaped thorns. The fruit peels, seeds, bark and oil are also used in traditional medicine to treat cholera. This tree attracts bees, particularly honeybees, for pollination.

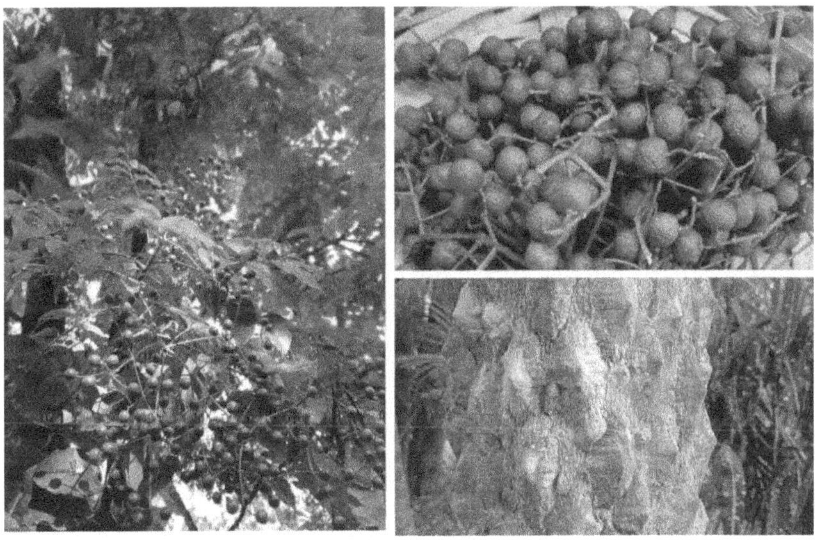

What is used - Various parts of the tree, including fruit peels, seeds, bark, and oil, are used in traditional medicines.

Propagation - Propagate through seed. Collect ripe berries, clean the seeds and stratify them before sowing. Root cuttings can be taken just after the rains and suckers can be separated from the base of mature plants.

Medicinal benefits

Toothache

The numbing effect caused by flower or husk extract helps to alleviate toothache by reducing the perception of pain signals. Chewing the plant's flowers or extracts can induce a numbing sensation that can last for up to 15 minutes. The plant has compounds which have anti-inflammatory effects and can reduce swelling and reddening associated to toothaches and other oral problems.

Immunity booster

The plant may also help boost the immune system. It contains compounds that are anti-bacterial, anti-fungal and anti-parasitic. Toothache Tree also has anti-microbial properties, which can help fight off infections in the mouth.

Dermatitis

Due to its anti-inflammatory properties, the toothache plant could relieve dermatitis. This condition occurs when the skin becomes inflamed and swollen.

Diuretic

The tropical plant is also a natural diuretic. Diuretics helps the body get rid of excess fluid by escessive urination.

Dry Mouth condition

The compound spilanthol in toothache tree stimulates salivary glands and prevents dry mouth and further and cracked lips.

The bark, fruit, and stem of the tree have been used in different forms, such as chewing, smoking and applying as a poultice.

51 Turmeric

Scientific name: *Curcuma longa*
In English: Turmeric
Konkani: Halad

Turmeric is a deep, golden-orange spice known for adding color, flavour and nutrition to foods. Turmeric powder is made from rhizomes of plants and has been used in cooking for hundreds of years in Goan kitchens.

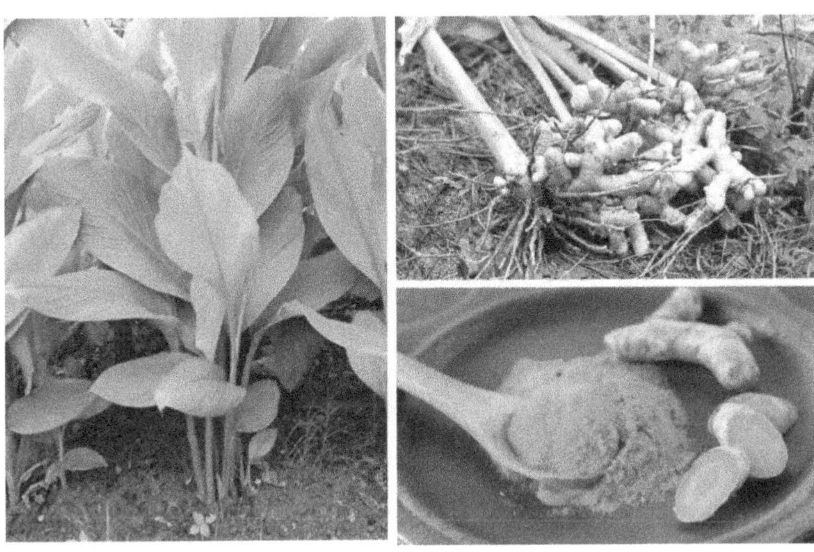

What is used - root

Propagation - To propagate turmeric, plant sections of the rhizome in well-drained and slightly alkaline soil. Ensure each piece of the rhizome has 2-3 buds, which can be sown 2 cm deep in soil.

Medicinal benefits

Improves body Immunity

Turmeric has anti-oxidant compounds, which help the body combat the damaging effects of a process called oxidation. Oxidation causes chronic inflammation and as a result, lead to conditions like heart disease, type 2 diabetes and cancer. When consumed at low doses, curcumin in turmeric enhances the antibody responses, helping fight off infection.

Taking turmeric may improve indigestion in some people.

Treating wounds from Infections

Traditionally, turmeric is also used as an antiseptic, for a cut or wound as it prevents infection. It also reduces the pain caused by the wound.

Improves Memory

A small amount of turmeric could even boost brain health. Reduction in brain inflammation and curcumin's anti-oxidant properties leads to less decline in neuro-cognition, the ability to think and reason.

Lower risk of Heart disease

Turmeric's ability to help reduce inflammation and oxidation, may lower the risk of heart disease. It also helps in reducing cholesterol.

Turmeric has a bitter taste and is frequently used to flavour or colour curry powders. It can be mixed in boiled raw milk for consumption to boost immunity.

52 Wild Karanda

Scientific name: *Carissa spinarum L.*
In English: Wild karanda
Konkani: Karvanda

Wild Karavanda is a medium sized thorny shrub and its fruit is small, succulent, fleshy and rounded with a juicy pulp. It is bitter-sour and acidic in taste and is popularly eaten directly while plucking from the plant. In Goa, it is now sold in markets or by the roadside, in a cone shaped banyan or jack fruit leaf. It's a good source of anti-oxidants, vitamins, and minerals, contributing to improved digestion, heart health, and immunity. Additionally, it's known for anti-inflammatory and anti-microbial properties.

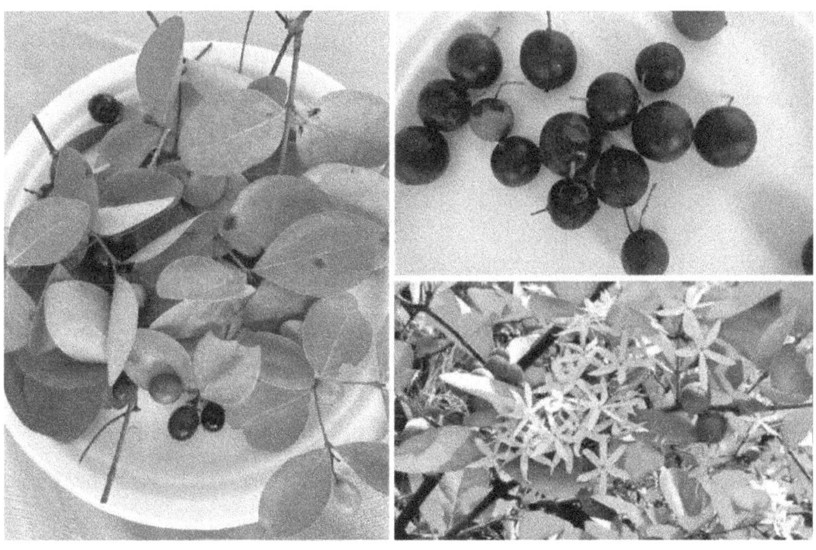

What is used - Fruit

Propagation -The plant is found in the wild in Goa. Propagation is mostly through seed and stem cutting, air layering and budding

Medicinal benefits

Helps in Digestion

Wild Karavanda is rich in fibre and water content, which can aid in digestion and relieve abdominal pain.

Good for the Heart

Wild Karavanda helps strengthen heart muscles, lower the risk of heart disease, and improve blood flow, due to its high potassium and anti-oxidant content.

Boost Immunity

Wild Karavanda high in Vitamin C content can boost the immune system, helping protect against common illnesses like cough, cold and viral fevers. Its anti-inflammatory properties can help reduce inflammation in the body, which is linked to various health conditions. Wild Karavanda contains various anti-oxidants, including flavonoids and phenolic compounds that can help in reducing oxidative stress and the risk of chronic heart diseases and cancer.

Mental Wellness

Magnesium, vitamins, and tryptophan in Wild Karavanda may contribute to improved mental health.

Blood Sugar Regulation

Wild Karavanda helps regulate blood sugar levels, which could be beneficial for diabetes.

Glossary

Anti-bacterial - destroying or stopping the growth of bacteria.

Anti-fungal - destroying or inhibiting the growth of fungus.

Anti-Inflammatory - controlling inflammation, a reaction to injury or infection.

Anti-microbial - active against microbes.

Antioxidant - prevents or inhibits oxidation.

Antiseptic - agent used to produce asepsis and to remove pus, blood, etc.

Antispasmodic - calming nervous and muscular spasms or convulsions.

Aphrodisiac - substance increasing capacity for sexual arousal.

Asthma - a respiratory condition marked by attacks of spasm in the bronchi of the lungs, causing difficulty in breathing.

Arthritis - disorder that affects joints and muscles.

Bronchitis - inflammation of the mucous membrane in the bronchial tubes.

Cardiotonic - increases strength and tone (response to stimuli) of the heart.

Carminative - causing the release of stomach or intestinal gas.

Carcinogenic - substance that causes cancer.

Chronic - a disease continuing for a long time.

Coma - the state of complete loss of consciousness

Constipation - is a condition in which there is difficulty in emptying the bowels.

Diarrhoea - loose motion.

Diuretic - increases flow of urine.

Eczema -common chronic skin condition characterized by dry, itchy, and inflamed skin.

Gingivitis - a common and mild form of gum disease, characterized by inflammation of the gums.

Hypertension - a fall in blood pressure below the normal level.

Insomnia - condition being unable to sleep.

Intoxication - a state of altered consciousness and behavior caused by the recent use of a psychoactive substance, such as alcohol or drugs

Laxative - having the action of loosening bowel.

Leprosy - discoloration and lumps on the skin and, in severe cases, disfigurement and deformities.

Migraine - a periodic condition with localised headaches, associated with vomiting and sensory disturbance.

Morbid - belonging or relating to disease.

Neuralgic - short, severe pains felt suddenly along a nerve, especially in the neck or head.

Paediatric - relating to the medical care of children.

Palpitation - fast and strong beating of the heart

Perspiration - the process of sweating.

Pneumonia - disease in which is linked to spongy tissue of the lung.

Prophylactic - prevention of development of disease.

Purgative - strongly laxative in effect.

Rheumatism - inflammation and pain in the joints.

Sinusitis - inflammation affecting the epithelium of a sinus.

Stimulant - a substance that raises levels of physiological or nervous activity in the body.

Trauma - a pathological alteration of the supporting tissues due to abnormal occlusion.

Tonsillitis - a painful infection of the tonsils.

Uteritis - inflammation of the uterus.

Refrences

Jain, S.K. 1975. Medicinal Plants. Thomson Press (India).

Mokat, D., Kharat, T.D. and Ade, A.B. 2025. Inspiring Stories in Medicinal Plants Sector (1st ed.). Pune, India: Regional-Cum-Faciliation Centre, Western Region Department of Botany, SPPU. ISBN: 978-93-342-3665-1.

Mokat, D.N. 2024. Medicinal Plants Wealth at Mahamana Vaidya Shankar Daji Shastri Pade - Medicinal Plants Garden (1st ed.). Pune, India: Savitribai Phule Pune University. ISBN: 9789334021530.